TIMES OF CRISIS

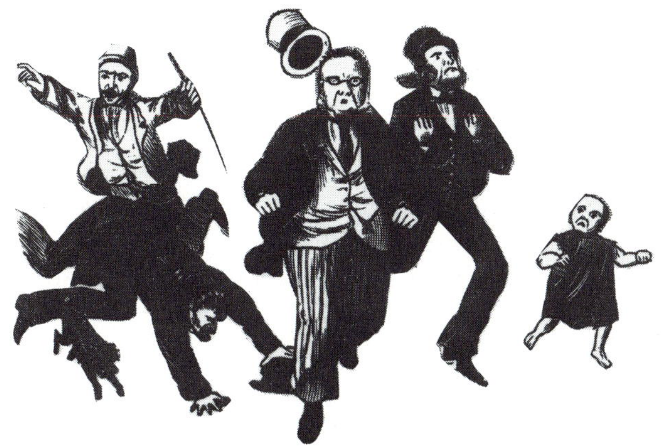

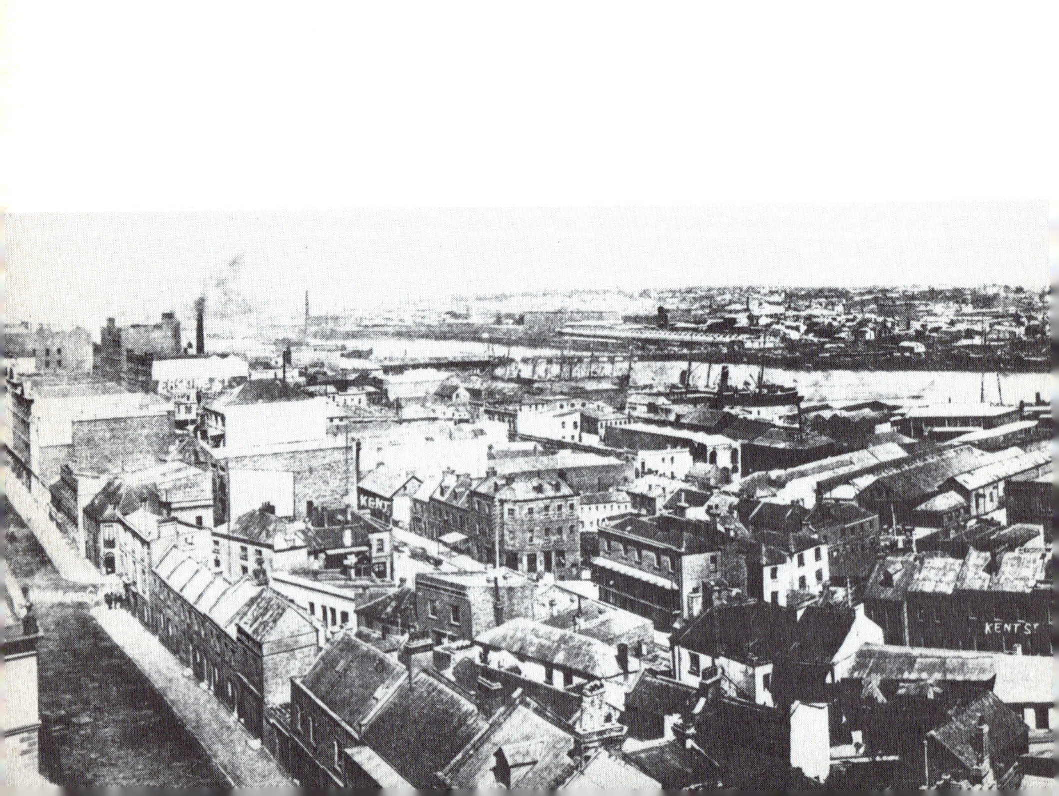
KENT
KENT ST

P. H. Curson

TIMES OF CRISIS

Epidemics in Sydney 1788–1900

Sydney University Press

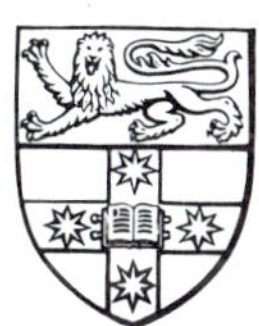

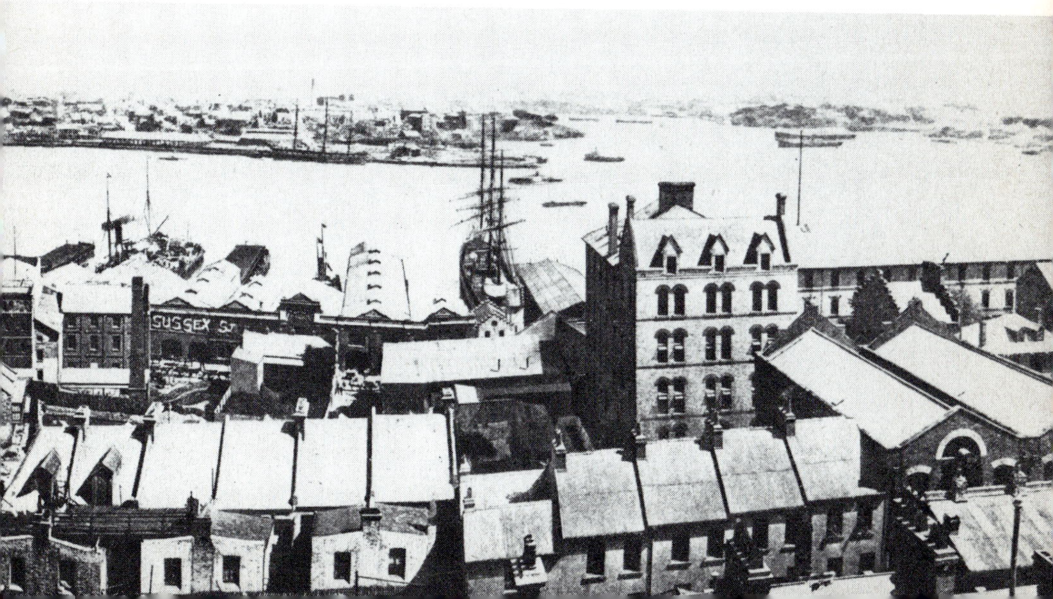

SYDNEY UNIVERSITY PRESS
Press Building, University of Sydney

UNITED KINGDOM, EUROPE, MIDDLE EAST, AFRICA
HB Sales, Enterprise House, Ashford Road
Ashford, Middlesex TW15 1XB, England
NORTH AND SOUTH AMERICA
International Specialized Book Services
P.O. Box 1632, Beaverton, Oregon 97075
United States of America

National Library of Australia Cataloguing-in-Publication data

Curson, Peter.
Times of crisis.

Bibliography.
Includes index.
ISBN 0 424 00112 8.

1. Epidemics — New South Wales — Sydney — History.
2. Public health — New South Wales — Sydney — History. I. Title.

614.4'994

Title page illustration
General view of quarantined and infected areas
around Darling Harbour in 1900.
(*Sydney Mail*, 31 March 1900. From the original in the
General Reference Library, State Library of
New South Wales)

First published 1985

Printed in Australia
by Macarthur Press Ltd, Parramatta

Contents

Illustrations

Photographs

Figures

ILLUSTRATIONS

Tables

Preface

THIS BOOK grew out of a desire to discover what were the effects of a number of traumatic epidemics of infectious disease that affected Sydney during the period 1788 to 1900. Although the six epidemics discussed in this book killed relatively few people they incapacitated many thousands and created an environment of bewilderment, panic and resentment. Given the recent resurgence of whooping cough and the upsurge of hysteria and panic surrounding AIDS (Acquired Immune Deficiency Syndrome) the reasons for my interest are obvious.

To a large extent this study depends upon material assembled from a wide array of unpublished sources mostly relating to death and disease. In particular, much use has been made of parish and cemetery burial records, official records of death and a variety of hospital and disease registers. The hazards of such an exercise stem in large part from the fact that I have had to rely heavily upon mortality rather than morbidity data. One of the basic problems inherent in the reconstruction of past epidemics is that in many cases such events have not left a clear record of cases as opposed to deaths. Consequently, while it is possible to reconstruct with some accuracy the deaths that occurred from particular epidemics we can only guess at the numbers who were affected but subsequently recovered. In the present study only in the case of the smallpox epidemic of 1881–2 and the plague outbreak of 1900 has it proved possible to assemble a list of those who caught the disease and survived. For the remaining four epidemics the discussion rests on the death record and to this extent the full impact of these disasters may be understated.

Much of the research on which this book is based was carried out in the office of the New South Wales Registrar-General, the Mitchell Library, the Archives Office of New South Wales, the Public Records Office, London as well as numerous church and parish offices. I would like to express my thanks to the staff of these institutions for their courteous and helpful assistance. In particular I am indebted to Mr Imrie of the Registrar-General's office for allowing me access to nineteenth-century death records, to the Rev. Fox, late of St Philips, for introducing me to that church's unmatched repository of parish registers, to Monsignor Duffy of St Mary's Cathedral for permission to consult Catholic archives, to the Rev. Austin Day of Christchurch St Lawrence and the Rev. Clout of Holy Trinity for permission to consult their early church registers. For assistance in the complexities of Aboriginal society and culture at the time of first settlement I am indebted to Anne Ross at Macquarie University. The chapter on plague owes much to my friendship and fruitful collaboration with Kevin McCracken and in particular our long-term large-scale study of this, the most fascinating of nineteenth-century epidemics. Considerable thanks are also due to John Cleasby and Rod Bashford for drafting all the diagrams and to Daisy Lee and Olga Zacroczymski for typing the manuscript. I also owe a considerable debt to Sam Fulton, Elizabeth Mitchell, Gail Hesselman, Angela Lindstadt and Jenny Rich for substantial research, and to Professor K. Cable of Sydney University for permission to copy his personal record of burials registered at St James Church.

The research on which this book is based was partly funded by the Australian Research Grants Committee and partly by Macquarie University. The first draft was written while I was on leave at the Centre for Population Studies, London School of Hygiene and Tropical Medicine. I thank the Director, Professor W. Brass, for his hospitality and kindness. My largest debt is to my wife, Sheila, for her help and encouragement. She deserves better acknowledgement than this book.

CHAPTER ONE

Introduction

DEATH AND DISEASE are only rarely a matter of chance. Rather they are invariably an expression of the way a population is organized socially and spatially, the stresses to which individuals are exposed, their genetic constitution, the vagaries of the physical environment and patterns of intercourse and mobility. Every society has to resolve the problem of the conflict between life and death and the place of disease. The nature of this problem and the way in which a society goes about solving it largely reflect the socio-cultural, economic, spatial and political way in which a society is organized together with the prevailing state of knowledge about death and disease. Death and disease should not be seen, therefore, as isolated considerations but as integral to the functioning of a society and part of the complex web of attitudes, beliefs and values that make up part of the culture of a society. Today, disease and illness are largely treated as natural phenomena amenable to scientific investigation. Prior to the latter part of the nineteenth century (and in parts of the underdeveloped world today), disease was seen as a manifestation of supernatural forces requiring causal explanations. The element of chance may have also played a more important role prior to the twentieth century. In societies where life expectancy was low and mortality, particularly infant mortality, high, where living and working conditions were hazardous and insanitary and where food and water were often polluted or contaminated, many children only survived to their teens if they were lucky. In the nineteenth century death and disease were conspicuous, regular and frequent companions of everyday life. Unlike our own society where death and disease have largely become confined to a handful of identifiable social groups (the elderly, the retired and the infirm) as well as the domain of specialized institutions largely removed from the routine of daily life, such societies had to incorporate the severity of death and disease into their everyday frame of living.

Throughout history, man has been both fascinated and repelled by the spectre of death and disease and by those dramatic confrontations with disaster where death or illness were the likely outcome. Such confrontations serve to remind us not only that we are mortal but also that we are frequently vulnerable to the vagaries of the biological environment. The greatest natural disasters of all time have been epidemics of infectious disease such as plague, smallpox, cholera, influenza and yellow fever. Periodic outbursts of such diseases exacted a fearful toll of human life and had a profound effect on the course of human events. The sheer magnitude of casualties from epidemic disease is staggering to behold and makes mortality from all other causes, natural or man-made, seem trivial in comparison. Thus in Europe during the fourteenth century plague caused some 25 million deaths out of the total population of 100 million (Bailey, 1975:3), and in the unsettled period between 1910 and 1921, whereas wars, revolution and massacres accounted for approximately 11.4 million deaths, epidemic disease carried off between 23 and 26 million (Bouthoul and Carrère, 1976).

EPIDEMICS

It has become conventional to distinguish between *endemic* diseases, which persist in a population over a prolonged time period, and *epidemic* diseases, which are seen as periodic invasions by a particular type of infectious agent resulting in a sudden explosive outburst of cases and deaths sharply concentrated in time and space. In many ways the distinction is unsatisfactory and it is probably better to make a broad distinction between *transmissable* diseases, which result from the invasion of a living stimulus such as a virus or bacteria, *degenerative* diseases, resulting largely from non-living stimuli, and *behavioural* diseases, resulting from psycho-social and environmental stress. If we adopt such a classification, then *endemic* and *epidemic* simply become terms of incidence and prevalence rather than signposts of particular diseases. The fact remains, however, that the term *epidemic* has a particular connotation in the popular mind, one associated with a specific state of being — something that comes upon a population from without and is prevalent for a limited period of time. The term *epidemic* also unfortunately lacks quantitative precision. In many ways epidemics are determined by the temporal and spatial frame in which they occur. For example, an epidemic may be considered to involve 15 cases of measles over a period of a few weeks in a small orphanage, 30 cases of typhoid in two months in a small town, 40 cases of food poisoning in a few hours on an international airliner or 2000 cases of influenza spread over four or five months in a large city. Further, in some cases it is not the impact of the agent in terms of cases or deaths or the temporal-spatial frame that is important so much as the public perception of and reaction to the disease involved. Thus a handful of plague or smallpox cases in a large city may be regarded as an epidemic simply because of the emotional reaction engendered by the disease. Epidemics are consequently multi-faceted phenomena distinguishable at least in the public eye not only in terms of their epidemiological impact (a series of cases and deaths concentrated in time-space) but also by the psycho-social reaction they engender. In all cases, however, epidemics represent a convergence in time and space of an infectious agent and a susceptible host as well as in some cases an intermediary vector.

This raises the question as to how best to define an epidemic. Should the criteria be primarily *epidemiological*, that is, numbers ill or dead or the impact on health care facilities? Should *social* criteria be considered, for example, when an outbreak of disease is sufficient to cause substantial disruption to the normal social and economic processes of daily life? Finally, should the criteria be *psycho-social*, where the nature of the disease involved is perceived to be such as to give rise to an outpouring of fear, anxiety and panic? Most of the literature on epidemic crises in the past relies on a strictly demographic definition usually searching out periods of exceptional mortality within some given time period. In addition, such work usually relates the period of exceptional mortality to some 'normal' experience of adjoining periods as well as considering the duration of the crisis and the size of the population involved (Hollingsworth, 1979). Clearly such considerations are important but they represent only one of a number of ways of defining an epidemic crisis. An epidemic would seem to be far more than a mere epidemiological or demographic event. Were it only that, the public would react with less drama. It would seem, therefore, that at least two sorts of epidemics exist, one defined principally in terms of the morbidity and/or mortality produced and the other in terms of the psycho-social reaction engendered.

Epidemics for the purpose of this present study are, therefore, defined as where an infectious disease agent produces an excess of illness or death in a restricted time-space framework and/or where the public reaction to the particular disease involved is sufficient to produce a marked reaction in attitudes and behaviour. The former could perhaps be labelled a *demographic crisis*, the latter a *crisis of confidence* or an epidemic in the *minds of the public*.

It would also seem that spatially and temporally there are at least two distinct types of epidemic. The first, *point* or *common-source* epidemics, are usually those most rigorously defined in time and space where a number of susceptible individuals are more-or-less simultaneously exposed to a common source of pathogenic infection, for example, holiday-makers onboard an ocean liner exposed to food contaminated with staphylococci. This type of exposure results in an explosive increase in the number of cases of disease in a restricted time-space framework. The second, *contagious* or *propagated* epidemics, result from the direct or indirect transmission of an infectious agent from one susceptible host to another. This can take place through direct person-to-person transmission or it can sometimes involve a more complex route in which the agent must pass through a vector.

In order to understand the nature of epidemics of infectious disease it is necessary to appreciate how infections spread through a population. Most of the acute infectious diseases responsible for major epidemics both in the past and today are spread in one of four ways.

1. *Airborne droplet infections*

Many of the more common infectious diseases such as measles, scarlet fever, influenza and whooping cough as well as diseases important in the past such as smallpox and pneumonic plague were transmitted directly from person to person via the medium of small droplets of saliva forcibly expelled during speech, sneezing or coughing and suspended in the air. In any confined living space, particularly in a moisture-laden atmosphere, such droplets may become suspended in the air to be inhaled by other persons present (Burnet and White, 1972:108). Even under the most favourable conditions epidemics of such diseases cannot occur unless a large proportion of the population is susceptible to infection. Whether an infectious agent spreads epidemically depends on the level of immunity present in a community, which normally reflects each individual's prior exposure to the particular infection and the duration of immunity conferred by a single attack. In some cases, such as measles and smallpox, a single exposure may be enough to confer life-long immunity; in others, such as influenza, the length of immunity is much shorter (Boycott, 1971:24–5). The spread of person-to-person infections is also influenced by human attitudes and decisions, particularly those relating to personal, spatial, social and economic behaviour. Such attitudes and decisions manifest themselves in spatial patterns of intercourse and movement, congregation and activities, at the local, regional and national level (Angulo *et al.*, 1979). The amount and nature of human social and spatial interaction is a crucial variable. Such interaction is usually governed by such factors as distance, the spatial distribution of attractions and facilities, and the kin and friendship network.

2. *Infections spread via food and water*
Human susceptibility is also an important factor in the second group of diseases, those spread in food and water. Faecal contamination of water, milk, foodstuffs and utensils provides a ready vehicle for the transmission of a number of important enteric infections, chief among which are cholera, typhoid fever, dysentery and diarrhoea. In addition, disease can arise from the contamination of foodstuffs by the salmonellae and shigella. Population crowding linked to marginal public health conditions including lack of hygiene and contamination of food and water supplies contribute markedly to the incidence of such infections.

3. *Infections spread by close bodily contact*
The sexually transmitted diseases are all spread by close bodily contact. Currently more than twenty different pathogens have been linked with such diseases. To a certain extent such diseases are also closely related to human crowding and behaviour in so far as their spread is often a function of proximity and increased sexual activity.

4. *Vector spread diseases*
There remains a number of infectious diseases which require the physical intervention of an intermediary or vector to act as the link in the chain of infection to humans. Normally such infections are transmitted to humans by the bite of insects. Malaria, bubonic plague, yellow fever, typhus and encephalitis all fall within this category.

THE GEOGRAPHY OF EPIDEMICS

The study of epidemics reveals them to be complex and fascinating phenomena with social and spatial implications well worthy of geographical investigation. In geographical terms an epidemic represents a convergence in time and space of an agent (sometimes also a vector) and a susceptible population involving sequences of socio-spatial interaction, action and reaction. For a long time epidemics were considered to be either small-scale clinical problems or temporal phenomena. Yet epidemics, particularly those of infectious disease, share the property of spatial diffusion and are particularly interesting for their ability to spread outwards or to disperse from one or more centres to other geographical areas (Cliff *et al.*, 1981:1). Considerable attention by geographers has in recent years been directed towards a search for spatial order in this diffusion process in the hope of comprehending and unravelling the mechanisms and processes involved. The geography of epidemics has thus tended to concentrate on the spatial aspects of infectious disease particularly with reference to their areal spread, although some attempts have also been made to understand more fully the nature of disease transmission and the environmental and socio-economic conditions that facilitate its appearance and spread. In many cases such studies have adopted an ecological framework. Integral to such an approach has been the assumption that diseases, like many other demographic and geographic phenomena, display distinctive areal distributional patterns and that geographical analysis is a useful and appropriate exercise which in some instances can illuminate underlying causes. In one or two cases geographers have also addressed the problem of modelling epidemics in human populations in an attempt to blend epidemiological and mathematical theory with that of spatial analysis. Haggett's modelling of measles epidemics in southwest England and Brownlea's development of a geographical model of infectious hepatitis are two examples of this approach (Haggett, 1972; Brownlea, 1972). A more recent study of the historical diffusion of measles epidemics in Iceland by Cliff *et al.*, reveals what can be achieved by an amalgamation of epidemiology, spatial diffusion theory, time series models and cartographic techniques (Cliff *et al.*, 1981).

An emerging area of geographical interest in recent years has been a concern with understanding the distribution of infectious disease in past populations and the nature of the spatial diffusion of historic epidemics. Ray, for example, has discussed the diffusion of diseases as a result of the nineteenth-century fur trade in Canada (Ray, 1976); Stock, the diffusion of cholera in West Africa (Stock, 1976); Pyle, the diffusion of cholera in nineteenth-century U.S.A. (Pyle, 1969); and more recently Morrill and Angulo have investigated the epidemic progression of an outbreak of smallpox (variola minor) in a small Brazilian city (Morrill and Angulo, 1979). Most of these studies have been concerned with the spatial impact of epidemic disease and its diffusion mainly at the local, regional, national and international level. Few attempts have been made to reconstruct attitudes and behaviour, to search out the psycho-social impact of particular epidemics or see such events as emotional and psychological phenomena (see, for example, Langer, 1958 and Baehrel, 1950). Historians have by contrast been much more concerned with reconstructing the socio-economic and political environment within which epidemics occur but in doing so have largely ignored consideration of the spatial consequences or diffusion patterns (see, for example, Alexander, 1980; Chevalier, 1958; Cooper, 1965; McGrew, 1965).

EPIDEMIC DISEASE IN THE NINETEENTH CENTURY

Today it is difficult to imagine a situation where people were continually confronted by the prospect of death or disfigurement stemming from epidemics of infectious disease over which they had little or no control. The prospect of sudden death from epidemics of infectious disease has largely faded away. Traffic accidents, cancer, heart attacks, stroke and venereal disease have to some extent taken its place but for the vast majority of people disease causing death or illness beyond a few days in bed with influenza simply no longer plays a major part in their life.[1] Not so during the nineteenth century, however, when death and disease were major preoccupations and where epidemics of infectious disease caused untold suffering. It is very difficult for us today to imagine the significance of disease as a constant companion of everyday life. In the nineteenth century minor irritations like dyspepsia, the common cold and toothache often assumed major proportions. Yet suffering seems to have been stoically borne, perhaps because it was so universal, so inevitable and because it affected most social groups (Eversley, 1965:35). Characteristically death and disease were regarded as commonplace and hardly mentioned unless they assumed catastrophic proportions. As Eversley points out,

> In the period where a third of all babies died before they were one year old . . . the loss of a small child can hardly have been treated as a major tragedy. When the expectation of life at birth for all people was between twenty and thirty years . . . the loss of a member of the family group was a constantly recurring event. (Eversley, 1965:35–6)

It is against this sort of background that one must examine the onset of epidemics in nineteenth-century Sydney.

Faced with outbreaks of disease people invariably react according to the prevailing attitudes regarding disease causation. Throughout most of the nineteenth century, epidemic diseases were referred to as *zymotic* diseases. *Zymotic* from the Greek *zymos* meant fermentation, and such diseases were believed to originate from the fermentation of the body's tissues produced by some external stimuli. Many diseases were thought to be harboured by poisonous substances emanating from the soil and given off as noxious emissions during periods of unfavourable climatic or seismic conditions. Such *miasma*, as they were called, were also produced by humans themselves, by the products of their households and by their domestic animals as well as by cosmic influences beyond their control. To the average person such visitations were seen more as the 'Wrath of God', divine retribution for man's sinfulness. Towards the end of the century the work of Pasteur and Lister established beyond a doubt that infectious and other diseases were due to living microscopic organisms, and in a few years the bacilli that caused typhoid, diphtheria and tuberculosis were identified and the relationship between polluted water and contaminated food and the occurrence of typhoid established. Yet by 1900 opinion was still divided in Sydney and many medical practitioners had not accepted the germ theory of infectious disease.

THE PRESENT STUDY

The present study examines the socio-geographic nature of a series of epidemics of infectious disease which affected Sydney between 1788 and 1900. The aim is to comprehend better the reasons why such epidemics occurred, their social and demographic impact, the mechanisms of their transmission, their spatial diffusion through the city and the attitudes and behaviour they produced.

[1] The pendulum is finely balanced, however. The recent epidemic of whooping cough in the United Kingdom and the periodic outbursts of influenza, although they may not kill as many people as formerly, still cause a great deal of concern and human suffering.

INTRODUCTION

The six epidemics to be examined occurred in Sydney in 1789, 1867, 1875–6, 1881–2, 1891 and 1900. All were traumatic events in Sydney's demographic and social history. The epidemic of 1789 remains the most problematical of the six. Was it smallpox that caused such devastation among the Aboriginal population in the vicinity of Sydney, or some other disease? If the contemporary accounts are anywhere near accurate in their assessment of this epidemic's effects then it is the only example of a major mortality crisis in Australian history comparable with some of the great mortality crises of the Old World. The 1867 measles epidemic represents a major childhood epidemic, possibly the greatest childhood epidemic ever to occur in Australia. The scarlet fever outbreak of 1875–6 was also an important childhood epidemic but it differed from the earlier measles epidemic in the reactions it provoked. Whereas measles was largely accepted as a normal event of childhood, scarlet fever was by contrast a much more dreaded disease and the epidemic produced considerable public reaction. It also produced the first hesitant steps in the formulation of an official policy designed to handle epidemics of infectious disease. The smallpox epidemic of 1881–2 represents the first major emotional upheaval associated with infectious disease during the nineteenth century. Although actual cases and deaths were few, the outbreak was the first in Sydney's history to evoke large-scale scenes of hysteria, fear and panic. It was natural in such circumstances that scapegoats should be sought, and a wave of reaction was directed against the city's Chinese community. The influenza epidemic of 1891 was the first time Sydney had been caught up in a major pandemic of infectious disease. It was also the first epidemic with widespread effects and few Sydney families escaped its ravages. Finally, the bubonic plague outbreak of 1900, like the earlier smallpox epidemic, produced incredible scenes of mass hysteria, panic and helplessness. Although deaths only amounted to 103, the epidemic caused widespread social and economic dislocation and was undoubtedly the greatest social upheaval of nineteenth-century Sydney.

The way in which Sydney prepared for and responded to these traumatic episodes of infectious disease provides us with an insight into prevailing social attitudes and patterns of association, activity and mobility, and reveals aspects of behaviour and social organization that otherwise might remain hidden. The psycho-social climate engendered by these epidemics also reveals many of the latent tensions and antagonisms that characterized nineteenth-century colonial society as well as demonstrating the strength and resilience of social and economic bonds.

The question might be asked, why concentrate on these epidemics when they did little to affect overall mortality and morbidity rates compared with the ravages of diseases such as diarrhoea, dysentery, tuberculosis, and their like?

In the words of Douglas Gordon, 'Man is always more impressed by the tempest than by the gentle rain' (Gordon, 1976:159). So it was with these six epidemics. While their demographic impact was limited they none the less had tremendous shock value, captured the popular imagination and demanded far more attention than a wide range of endemic diseases which were responsible for sustaining high morbidity and mortality rates in Sydney. The symptoms of these diseases were one source of terror, their unpredictable geographic progress another. Plague and smallpox could, for example, creep silently along the back alleys or race swiftly across broad expanses of the city, leapfrogging whole streets and suburbs only in some cases to return at a later date. This study seeks, therefore, to explore the social and spatial aspects of these traumatic occurrences, and in particular community anxiety about public health and infectious disease. By way of introduction the work is prefaced by a broad overview of death and disease patterns during the period 1788–1900.

CHAPTER TWO

Disease and Death in Sydney

PATTERNS OF DISEASE

THE HISTORY OF INFECTIOUS DISEASE IN SYDNEY

The history of infectious disease in Sydney is a story of periodic waves rising and falling with the ebb and flow of immigration and economic fortune. In some cases, particularly after 1838, there were explosive epidemics of infectious disease with high case fatality rates. Always, however, such periodic outbursts were played out against a backdrop of a high incidence and prevalence of endemic debilitating diseases and although the pestilential diseases and childhood epidemics such as smallpox, plague, influenza and scarlet fever were held in great horror by the population, the real enemies which produced the highest morbidity and mortality throughout the nineteenth century were a series of less visible, more insidious diseases such as gastroenteritis, dysentery, diarrhoea, bronchitis, tuberculosis, venereal disease and a variety of eye and skin infections. It would appear that before 1820 most of the major infective diseases of childhood were unknown in the colony. One of the main reasons advanced for this was Australia's isolation in time and space from the major Old World sources of infection (see Young, 1979:214). Yet while it is true that many common infections failed to survive the long sea journey and burnt themselves out as localized shipboard infections it would really appear to have been the small and dispersed nature of Sydney's and New South Wales's population and the low proportion of young children which acted as a barrier against major outbreaks of infectious disease. Prior to the 1830s, if an infection did manage to survive the long sea journey, once on land it was generally short-lived and self-limiting owing to the small number of susceptibles and the dispersed nature of settlement.

Throughout the first 112 years of Sydney's development, infectious disease remained the handmaiden of immigration. In the period prior to 1815 the incidence of disease and the public health situation of the small town were very closely related to the arrival of convict transports and the transfer of ill and debilitated convicts to land. As well, the first two years of Sydney's life were a constant struggle for survival, aggravated by shortages of food and water and the unfamiliar environment. The history of enteric infections is closely associated with overcrowded and unhygienic conditions aboard convict and passenger ships and relates very closely to the two most important periods of immigration in New South Wales's history, 1790–1815 and 1838–60. The arrival of the Second and Third Fleets between 1790 and 1791 vividly illustrates not only the effect of high shipboard mortality and the landing of many ill convicts but also how this experience could remàin with the survivors and in some cases effectively shorten their lives. Both fleets suffered an appalling mortality and landed many convicts in a weak and sickly state. Of the 1243 convicts embarked in England aboard the Second Fleet, 272 or 22 per cent perished on the voyage and they were joined within twelve months of arrival by another 121. Of the 971 who were fortunate enough to survive the journey, over half were sick when the fleet arrived in Sydney. The transport *Neptune* suffered the heaviest mortality. Of the 502 convicts she embarked, almost one-third did not live to see Sydney, and of the 344 who did, 269 or 78 per cent were in such a perilous state of health as to raise serious doubts as to their continued survival. By mid-July 1790, 488 people were under medical treatment in the small settlement (Collins, 1971:103) and as Gandevia points out the high mortality which prevailed was largely confined to those who had arrived on the vessels of the Second Fleet (Gandevia and Cobley, 1974:115 and 121). The Third Fleet, which arrived a year or so later, also suffered considerable mortality. Of the 1695 males and 168 females embarked, 194 males and four females perished on the voyage and many of those landed were in a sickly and emaciated state. Seven months later Phillip could still report that many of those who had arrived were still in a weak and sickly state and that 288 had died since arrival (Cumpston, 1927:37). Although there is insufficient evidence to establish conclusively the nature of the disease or diseases responsible for such havoc there seems little doubt that scurvy, dysentery and typhus were mainly involved.

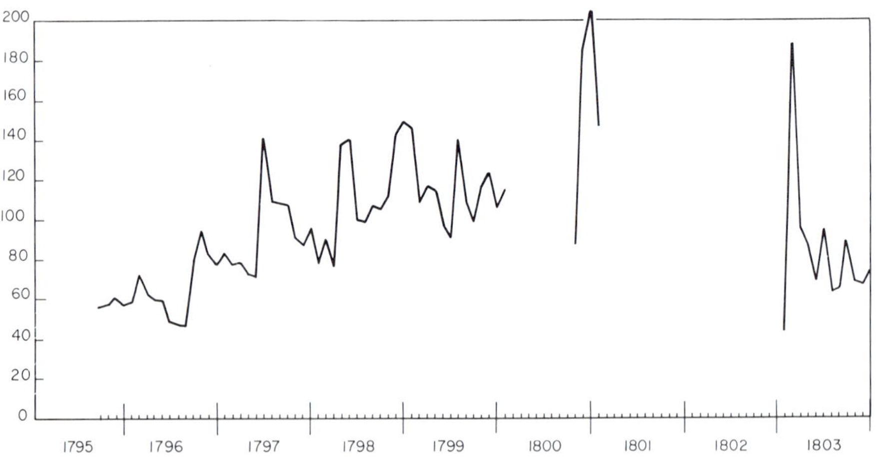

Figure 1 Monthly totals of sick 1795–1803

After the arrival of the Third Fleet, Sydney's general health situation seems to have greatly improved. Figure 1 details the monthly totals of persons sick in the town in the period between September 1795 and January 1800 and for a short period between 1800 and 1803. Even in relatively good times the arrival of an infected ship could quickly upset the balance of health in the town. For example, the two convict transports *Albion* and *Hillsborough* arrived in Sydney in late June 1799 having embarked 300 convicts in England. Both vessels suffered considerable mortality on the voyage to the extent that only 205 of the original contingent survived to make landfall (*HRA* I, 2:376) and many of these ended up in the hospital owing to widespread gaol fever, dysentery and scurvy. The figures for the number of persons sick in the town are missing from February to October 1800 but once again the November and December figures reveal just what impact the arrival of an ill-fated ship meant to Sydney's health situation. The *Royal Admiral* arrived in Sydney in late November 1800 after a severe outbreak of fever on the voyage. Between 43 and 49 convicts (the records quote both figures) were lost and of those landed many were very ill. Even two years later Governor King could draw attention to the fact that many convicts off the *Royal Admiral* remained in a debilitated state (*HRA* I, 2:697). Despite growing official concern at the excessive mortality and conditions aboard the transports the pattern recurred time and time again between 1800 and 1815. The *Atlas* and *Hercules* arrived within two weeks of each other in late June/early July 1802. Together they had embarked 320 convicts for New South Wales. Some convicts were apparently ill at the time of embarkation and during the voyage severe outbreaks of scurvy and dysentery carried off 127 convicts (almost 40 per cent!). Many of the survivors were in a dreadful state and even three months later were still in 'a state of convalescence, but too weak and debilitated to be ever of much use' (*HRA* I, 4:839).

After 1814 the health of the town returned to a more normal pattern of high levels of chronic disease. The daily record and outpatient registers of the Sydney Hospital for the period 1817–19 support the view that there was a high level of disease among the Sydney community. Data for a one-month period in 1819 show the majority of cases receiving treatment to have been people suffering from a variety of skin diseases (mainly ulcers and abscesses). Accidents and violence were next in importance, followed by venereal disease, catarrh and dysentery. In total these five groups accounted for more than 71 per cent of all cases under treatment (Table 1). The period between 1815 and 1836 seems to have been marked by a high level of dysentery and other gastrointestinal disorders as well as a variety of skin, eye and venereal diseases, catarrh, and a high level of accidents and violence. A number of contemporary observers drew attention to the high level of chronic disease. Lesson, the second surgeon aboard a French ship that visited Sydney in 1824, left us the following account about Sydney's health condition:

> The illnesses most common . . . are abdominal and pulmonary complaints. The former arise from faulty diet and alcoholic excesses to which a large part of the population is given . . . gastritis and enteritis are very frequent, but particularly hepatitis. . . . Dysentery . . . is prevalent in the summer. (quoted in Royle, 1973:951)

Cunningham, writing a year or two later, describes much the same pattern:

Table 1 Major Cases under Treatment, Sydney Hospital, 31 August–30 September 1819

Dislocations	8	Cynanche	12
Wounds[a]	67	Cephalalgia	17
Ulcers	236	Debility	15
Abscesses[b]	105	Lumbago	14
Contusions	81	Rheumatism	7
Dysentery	49	Pneumonia	13
Diarrhoea	5	Scrofula	11
Catarrh	61	Fontanelle	13
Constipation	22	Ophthalmia	10
Gonorrhoea[c]	64	Fever	3
Syphilis	19		

Source: Sydney Hospital, Day Books, 1817–19.
[a] Includes 18 related to flogging.
[b] Includes bubos, phlegmon, eruptions.
[c] Includes 3 other venereal.

Intermittents, remittents, typhus, scarlet fever, smallpox, measles, whooping cough, and croup are here unknown. . . . Dysentery is the most prevalent and fatal disease . . . yet deaths . . . from this cause are exceeding rare among the sober-living portion of the community, and far from common even among the debauched with whom dropsical affections are somewhat frequent. . . . Dyspeptic complaints are generally aggravated in the low, warm, portions of our country. . . . Children are very subject to the *teres*, or round-worm . . . and on reaching the age of puberty, phthisis is liable to supervene. . . . An epidemic influenza carried off a number of old Europeans some years ago. . . . This year [1826] it has again fatally visited the colony. An inflammation of the eyes, called 'the blight', often follows too. . . . True syphilis among the whites . . . appears to be unknown, but gonorrhoea is exceedingly common, and very virulent while it lasts. (Cunningham, 1966:94–5)

Reviewing the period between 1819 and 1836 Watson writes:

Dysentery remained the most prevalent disease. . . . of other diseases . . . rheumatism, venereal disease and 'dropsy' were almost as common. An annual cycle of ailments was observed: in the summer months, erysipelas was prevalent, especially among the young; in November, December and January, ophthalmia, taking chiefly the form of simple conjunctivitis . . . while in July, August and September, simple continued fever used to attack chiefly old people and children. In July and August 1820, an 'epidemic catarrh' raged throughout the Colony . . . and a second epidemic . . . reoccurred in November, 1825.[1] In 1824 mumps was epidemic. . . . In 1825 intermittent fever first appeared and in March, 1828, whooping cough was epidemic. (Watson, 1911:40 and 65)

1834–1900: THE ERA OF CHILDHOOD INFECTIONS

Although there had been isolated outbreaks of infectious disease during the 1820s it was not until the mid-1830s that the major childhood infections began to establish themselves in the town. Their appearance was undoubtedly related to the increase in shipping contacts and the rapid increase in immigration. The rise in importance of periodic epidemics of infectious disease should not, however, dis-

[1] This is an error on Watson's part. There is no record of unusual mortality in November 1825 in Sydney's burial records, yet for November 1826 deaths were considerably in excess of the average for previous and ensuing years.

guise the fact that Sydney's health situation continued throughout the nineteenth century to be dominated by a wide range of endemic diseases which took a heavy toll of life. Like the early period of Sydney's development such epidemics were intimately linked to immigration, although in this case free migrants rather than convicts. From the mid-1830s the history of infectious disease reveals a number of recurring themes: importation by ship from the Old World; dissemination throughout the urban community largely by personal contact; lack of effective means of control or treatment; a cyclical pattern of occurrence, lull and recurrence with particular diseases establishing a distinctive periodicity; and finally, a high incidence of such diseases amongst Sydney's poorer classes, leading to distinctive spatial concentrations of disease. From the mid-1830s there were growing reports of major outbreaks of the more common infectious diseases of childhood. Measles was one of the earliest diseases to appear. Although there had been cases of the disease reported aboard ships arriving at Sydney as early as 1829, the first major outbreak did not occur until 1834–5, probably introduced by the ship *David Scott* (see Donovan, 1970:5–10). Outbreaks of influenza and whooping cough followed in 1838–9, scarlet fever in 1840–1 and chickenpox in 1844. By the mid- to late 1840s, all these diseases had become well acquainted with the city and had

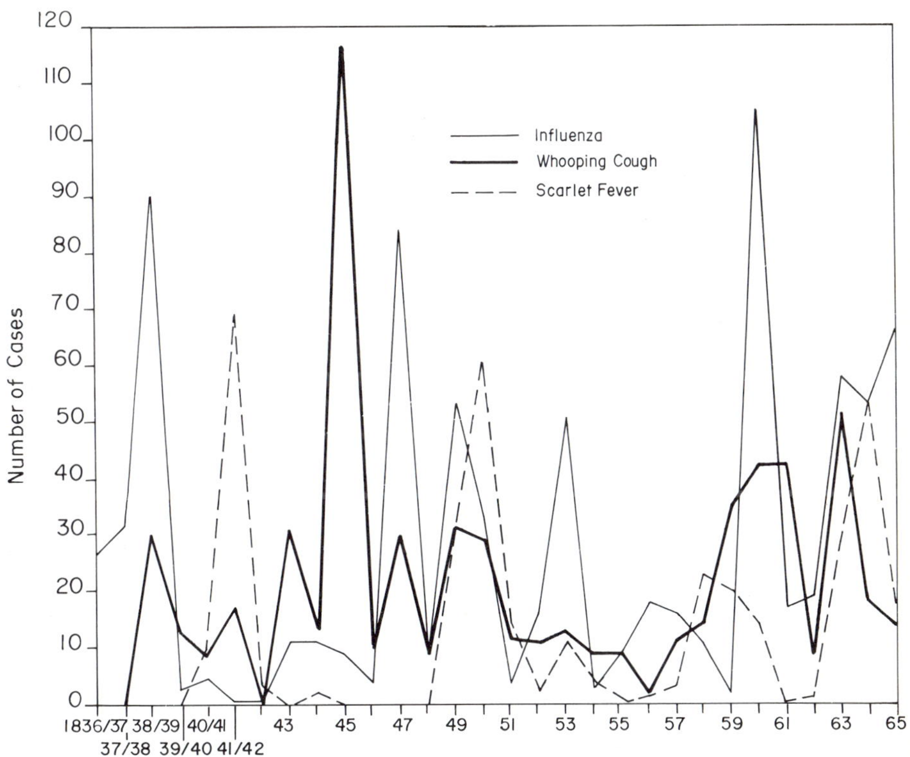

Figure 2 Cases of infectious disease, Sydney Dispensary/Infirmary 1836–65

adopted a regular cycle of occurrence and recurrence. Even at this early date the town could be swept up in pandemics of infectious disease imported from the Old World. The outbreaks of influenza in 1836–8, 1847 and 1850 are the first recorded occasions in which Australia shared in a pandemic of infectious disease. Figure 2 illustrates that between 1836 and 1865 influenza, whooping cough and scarlet fever adopted a wave-like periodicity with intervals between epidemic peaks varying from two to ten years. Such a pattern was to remain until at least the end of the century. The history of measles differs somewhat from the other major childhood infections. Although Sydney experienced an epidemic in 1834–5 it was not until 1853–4 that the next major outbreak occurred and the disease gained a firm foothold in the town. More population-size dependent than many other infections, measles requires a population in excess of 250 000 in order to survive and spread. In the case of Sydney, the disease had to await the 1850s and the explosive increase of population associated with the gold rushes. Once established in the town, it began a long-term association and epidemics occurred with a regular periodicity of five to eight years.

In many ways the period 1838–50 stands out as an important watershed in Sydney's socio-demographic and epidemiological development. Prior to this period the town languished as a small isolated convict outpost with an unbalanced age and sex ratio. The period between 1838 and 1850 changed all that. The dramatic increase in free migration followed by the discovery of gold during the 1850s transformed the town from a sleepy colonial outpost of 12 000 people to a bustling mercantile city of more than 50 000. Moreover, immigration, particularly of young families, radically altered the age and sex structure of the urban population. Whereas children under the age of 12 had comprised barely 20 per cent of the population before 1840, by 1851 they accounted for 30 per cent and by 1861 even more. Equally dramatic was the increase in the number of women. From a ratio of two males to one female in 1830 the figure had approached parity by 1850. With an increase in potential marriage partners the number of single adult males in the population declined substantially between 1830 and 1851. Such demographic changes provided the necessary base for the establishment of a wide range of childhood diseases by providing a large pool of susceptible children.

The arrival of large numbers of free immigrants in the ten years after 1838 had profound consequences for Sydney's public health. In the first place the incidence of infectious disease paralleled the increase in shipping arrivals. In the second, the increase in the number of young families and the continued high fertility created a rapidly expanding pool of young susceptibles. Conditions on board many of the immigrant ships were reminiscent of those during the convict period. Overcrowding was common, living conditions damp and unventilated and water and food supplies limited and monotonous. In addition, many passengers were embarked suffering from a variety of infectious diseases. Small wonder that mortality on the outward voyage was often substantial and that many made landfall suffering from a variety of diseases. Children died more readily than adults, usually from scarlet fever, whooping cough, measles, diphtheria, dysentery and typhoid. The experience of the *Beejapore* in 1852 was fairly typical. A transport of 1672 tons, she left England for Sydney with 1023 passengers and 40 crew. During her 85-day passage the ship suffered outbreaks of measles and scarlet fever which resulted in 56 deaths, the majority children. On arrival in Sydney, 84 cases were still under treatment and the ship was quarantined for a period of 54 days. During this time another 68 passengers died. In the ten years after 1838 more than 120 000 immigrants arrived in Sydney, the majority in the period 1838–41. Against such a tide of new arrivals the colony's quarantine laws were totally inadequate. Framed in 1832 (and subsequently amended to 1853) to deal only with maritime quarantine and not indigenous cases of disease, these laws represented a slavish copy of their English counterparts and were initially inspired by the fear of cholera. From 1841 the act empowered the Health Officer of Port Jackson to inspect all newly arrived vessels and from 1853 required the ship's master to provide written details of any shipboard illnesses or deaths. In practice, however, many conspired to conceal such cases so as to avoid unnecessary delay.

If Sydney's population had increased rapidly between 1830 and 1850 it positively burgeoned in the next two decades. By 1861 more than 96 000 lived in the metropolitan area and ten years later almost 138 000. At the same time the proportion of the population living in the central city area (mainly the City of Sydney) began to decline steadily as transport improved and new suburbs opened up. Rapid urbanization brought back old diseases. Overcrowding, poor sanitation, contaminated food and polluted water saw typhoid and a variety of enteric diseases become much more prevalent and a common cause of death. Deaths from dysentery, diarrhoea and enteritis increased precipitously in the fifteen years after 1850 and remained a major cause of death and disease at least until the end of the century.

The annual records of cases treated at the Sydney Dispensary and Infirmary provide some information on the town's health situation between 1836 and 1865.[2] Figure 3, which indicates the number of cases treated per 1000 population, suggests a fairly high level of ill-health in Sydney, particularly in the period 1836–51. When individual groups of diseases are examined they reveal much the same picture (Figures 4 and 5). What stands out, however, is that although episodes of infectious disease were often calamitous and shattering in their impact, it was the lesser, more ubiquitous diseases such as gastrointestinal disorders (dyspepsia, constipation) and skin diseases (ulcers, abscesses, boils, erysipelas) which dominated the everyday health scene. In times of severe economic hardship such as occurred in 1841–3 health conditions could deteriorate further so as to produce a surge in the number of people suffering from gastrointestinal disorders (Figure 6). Throughout this 30-year period disease patterns exhibited a certain degree of continuity. This is borne out by the data in Table 2, which lists the ten leading diseases treated at the Dispensary/Infirmary for five periods between 1838 and 1881, and by Figure 7 which assesses the importance of individual groups of diseases relative to all diseases.

Between 1835 and 1880 the main scourges of Sydney's population were the childhood infections scarlet fever, measles, whooping cough and diphtheria as well as a number of enteric diseases. From 1870 such diseases were joined by another group, tuberculosis (phthisis), smallpox, influenza, typhoid, and most ominously

[2] Information is also available for the Benevolent Asylum, but the returns are either too fragmentary or do not coincide with the same time period as the Dispensary.

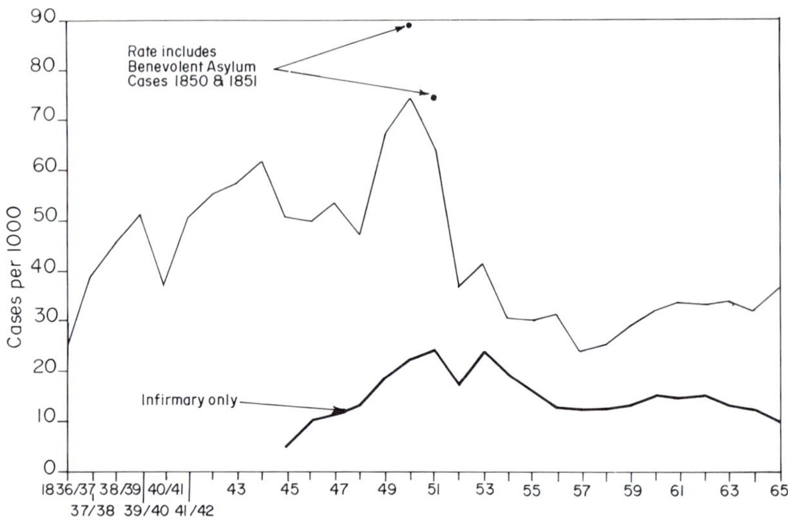

Figure 3 Total cases per 1000, Sydney Dispensary/Infirmary 1836–65

of all, bubonic plague. The rapid rise of industry and noxious trades in the town also exposed many urban dwellers to a variety of occupational risks and hazards. After 1840 the proliferation of slaughterhouses, boiling-down works, fellmongers, tallow and rope manufacturers, woolscourers, bone mills and tanneries greatly contributed to environmental pollution and the dissemination of infectious disease. The differentiation of trades and the occupational hazards associated with particular activities also began to have a detrimental effect on the health of Sydney's workers. The adverse effects of lead, mercury and arsenic poisoning became noticeable from at least the late 1830s. Lead poisoning in particular seems to have been responsible for a high level of sickness in the 1850s and 1860s. Between 1860 and 1865, for example, 243 people were treated for lead poisoning at the Sydney Dispensary and Infirmary. Many cases undoubtedly stemmed from contamination of the city's water supply by use of lead pipes and roofing. Others arose from the widespread practice of using lead as a colouring in foodstuffs. Employees in foundries, painting and plumbing works were particularly at risk. Cases of mercury poisoning were also widespread in the period 1840–70 as indeed were cases of arsenic poisoning. In the latter case the widespread use of arsenic as a pigment in many wallpapers as well as an important ingredient in a variety of sheepdip and vermin mixes explains its widespread prevalence (see Gandevia, 1971).

From the mid-1870s the threat of epidemic disease began to provoke middle-class concern for sanitary reform and public health. The scarlet fever outbreak of 1875–6, the smallpox epidemic of 1881–2 and the typhoid outbreaks of 1885–6 brought a new awareness of living conditions, urban sanitary conditions and public health. A Health Society of New South Wales was formed in 1876 primarily as a middle-class movement for sanitary reform. The 1880s marked the real begin-

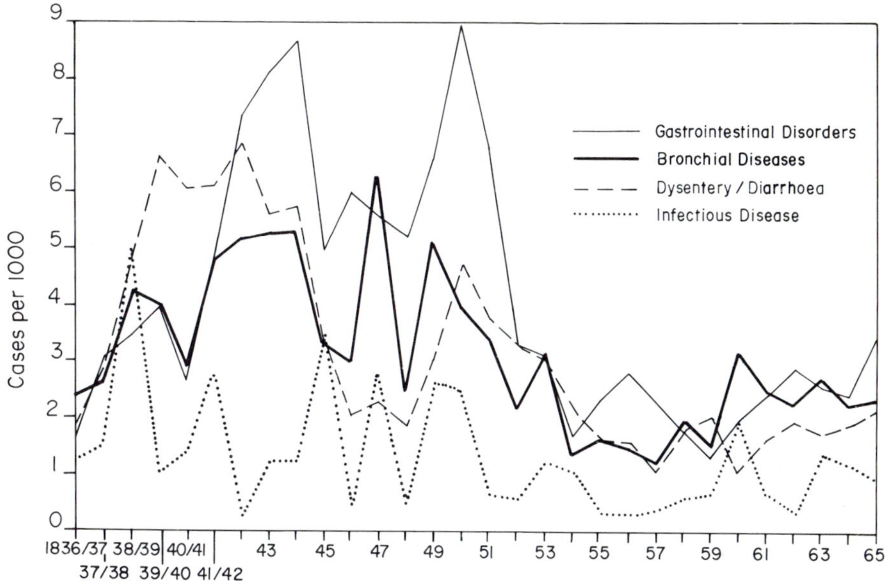

Figure 4 Cases per 1000, selected groups of diseases, Sydney Dispensary/Infirmary 1836–65

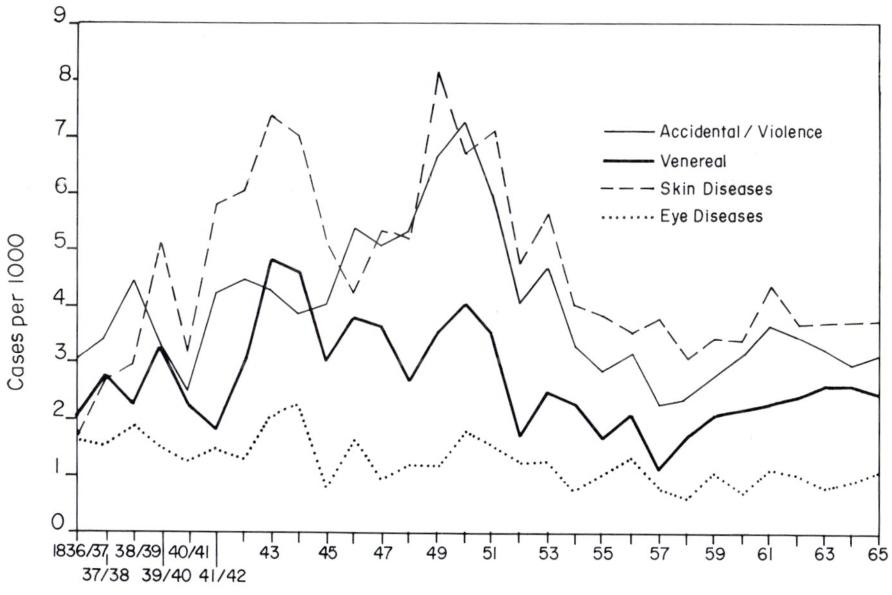

Figure 5 Cases per 1000, selected groups of diseases, Sydney Dispensary/Infirmary 1836–65

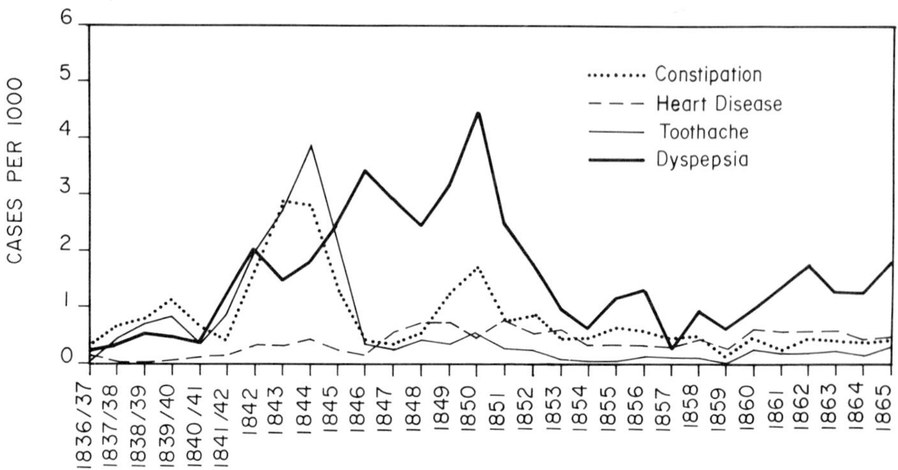

Figure 6 Cases per 1000, gastric disorders and heart disease, Sydney Dispensary/Infirmary 1836–65

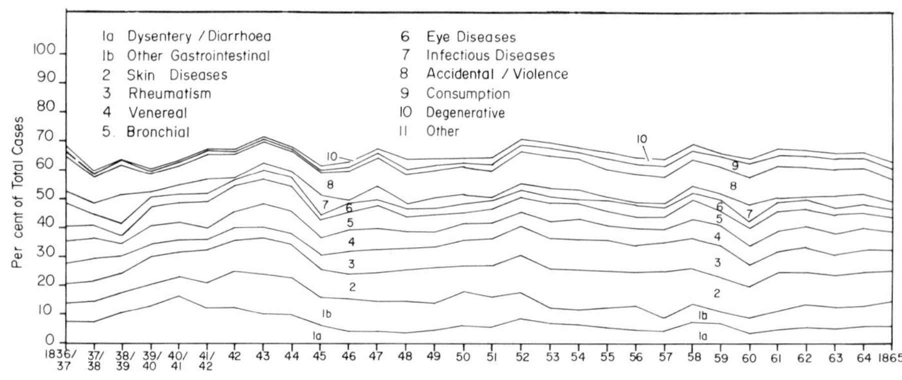

Figure 7 Diseases treated at Sydney Dispensary/Infirmary 1836–65

nings of public health legislation. As a result of the smallpox epidemic of 1881–2 an Infectious Diseases Act was passed in 1882 requiring the notification and registration of all smallpox cases. A Central Board of Health was also established and a Medical Adviser to the government, to oversee public health matters particularly in Sydney. The Coast Hospital was established as an isolation hospital with particular concern for infectious diseases and the Quarantine Station at North Head was organized on more formal lines providing short-term accommodation for cases of infectious disease. The 1880s and 1890s also saw considerable improvement in the city's drainage and sewerage system as well as legislation regulating the removal of nightsoil, the supervision of milk products, the prevention of nuisances

Table 2 Ten Leading Diseases Treated at Sydney Dispensary and Infirmary, 1838–9, 1849, 1859, 1874, 1881

Rank	*Disease* 1838–9	*% of total cases*	*Rank*	*Disease* 1849	*% of total cases*
1	Accidents/violence	9.6	1	Accidents/violence	9.9
2	Influenza	7.4	2	Rheumatism	7.0
3	Diarrhoea	5.8	3	Ulcers	6.2
4	Rheumatism	5.7	4	Venereal	5.2
5	Dysentery	4.9	5	Dyspepsia	4.7
6	Venereal	4.8	6	Inflammation of bronchia	3.6
7	Ulcers	3.8	7	Diarrhoea	2.6
8	Inflammation of eye	3.7	8	Abscess	2.0
9	Whooping cough	2.5	9	Dysentery	1.9
10	Worms	2.2	10	Constipation	1.8
	1859			1874	
1	Rheumatism	11.2	1	Accidents/violence	20.0
2	Accidents/violence	9.3	2	Venereal	6.5
3	Venereal	7.0	3	Rheumatism	6.2
4	Diarrhoea	6.0	4	Phthisis	3.6
5	Ulcers	5.8	5	Bronchitis	3.1
6	Inflammation of bronchia	3.8	6	Typhoid	2.8
7	Phthisis	3.2	7	Dyspepsia	2.6
8	Inflammation of eye	2.7	8	Bright's disease	2.6
9	Dyspepsia	2.2	9	Epilepsy	2.5
10	Dysentery	1.5	10	Cancer	2.3
	1881				
1	Accidents/violence	25.5			
2	Rheumatism	6.9			
3	Alcoholism	5.1			
4	Phthisis	4.4			
5	Venereal	3.8			
6	Typhoid	3.0			
7	Pneumonia	2.8			
8	Disease of cord	2.2			
9	Bright's disease	2.0			
10	Bronchitis	1.9			

Source: Sydney Dispensary/Infirmary, *Annual Reports*.

and the location of noxious industries. Finally in 1898 a new Public Health Act became law, providing local municipalities with the authority to undertake surveys of housing conditions as well as to cleanse and disinfect premises thought to be dangerous to human health or implicated in the spread of infectious disease. Property owners could also be called upon, under threat of prosecution, to remedy any drainage, structural or sanitation faults. The new act also made the notification of a range of infectious diseases compulsory.

The late nineteenth century saw the continuation of the cycle of childhood epidemic diseases as well as the intrusion of such diseases as typhoid, influenza, smallpox and bubonic plague. Smallpox and plague fall into a class of their own.

Between 1877 and 1900 there were three outbreaks of smallpox in Sydney, culminating in the epidemic of 1881–2 which produced 163 cases and 41 deaths. The last decade of the nineteenth century saw Sydney caught up in two pandemics of Old World diseases. In 1890–1 Sydney was involved in the first major pandemic of influenza for 30 years, and in 1900 the pandemic of bubonic plague which swept out of China in 1894 engulfed the city.

SPATIAL PATTERNS OF DISEASE

Throughout the nineteenth century disease displayed distinctive areal distribution patterns within Sydney. It is, however, not possible to obtain any detailed information until the last decade of the century. The distribution of typhoid fever cases in 1894 is shown in Figure 8. Classically this infectious disease was associated with contaminated water and food supplies and its spatial distribution was indicative of poor or inadequate sanitary arrangements. In 1894 there were more than 600 cases of typhoid in Sydney, the majority concentrated in a broad belt stretching from Woolloomooloo through Surry Hills, Redfern, Chippendale and Darlington to Newtown via Camperdown. From Newtown the disease also extended in a northwesterly direction to Annandale and Leichhardt as well as southwesterly to St Peters and Marrickville. Finally there was a cluster of cases at Botany to the south (Figure 8). Figure 9, which shows the distribution of the average number of cases of infectious disease per 1000 population in 1898–1900, provides an overall view of the spatial pattern of disease at the end of the nineteenth century.[3] The areas of greatest risk were Botany and St Peters in the south, Willoughby to the north, and Concord, Burwood and Enfield in the west of the urban area. Suburbs lowest at risk were generally areas of high social class such as Vaucluse and Woollahra or areas of recent or peripheral settlement such as Drummoyne and Hurstville.

PATTERNS OF MORTALITY

Throughout the period 1788 to 1900 epidemics of infectious disease played a major role in the life and death struggle of Sydney's inhabitants. The principal features of mortality over this period were high death rates, dramatic short-lived fluctuations declining in severity towards the end of the century, high infant and child mortality particularly after 1830, and finally a steady decline in mortality towards the end of the century. The mortality profile (Figure 10) indicates that the death rate varied according to the influence of epidemics of infectious disease, immigration, economic fortune and public health developments.[4] This material vividly illustrates the wide fluctuations associated with the early convict period and at a later date with outbreaks of epidemic disease. Crucial to an understanding of these mortality fluctuations was the role of immigration, not only because it was the means by which new infections gained entry to the city but also because continued immigration radically changed the city's demographic and social structure. Epidemics were not the only reason for high mortality, however, and much of the

[3] The diseases in question were scarlet fever, diphtheria, typhoid and plague. Together these four diseases were responsible for 584 deaths and 7702 cases between 1898 and 1900.

[4] This mortality profile is based partly on unpublished parish and cemetery burial registers (1788–1856) and partly on official vital statistics from the Registrar-General's returns (1857–1900).

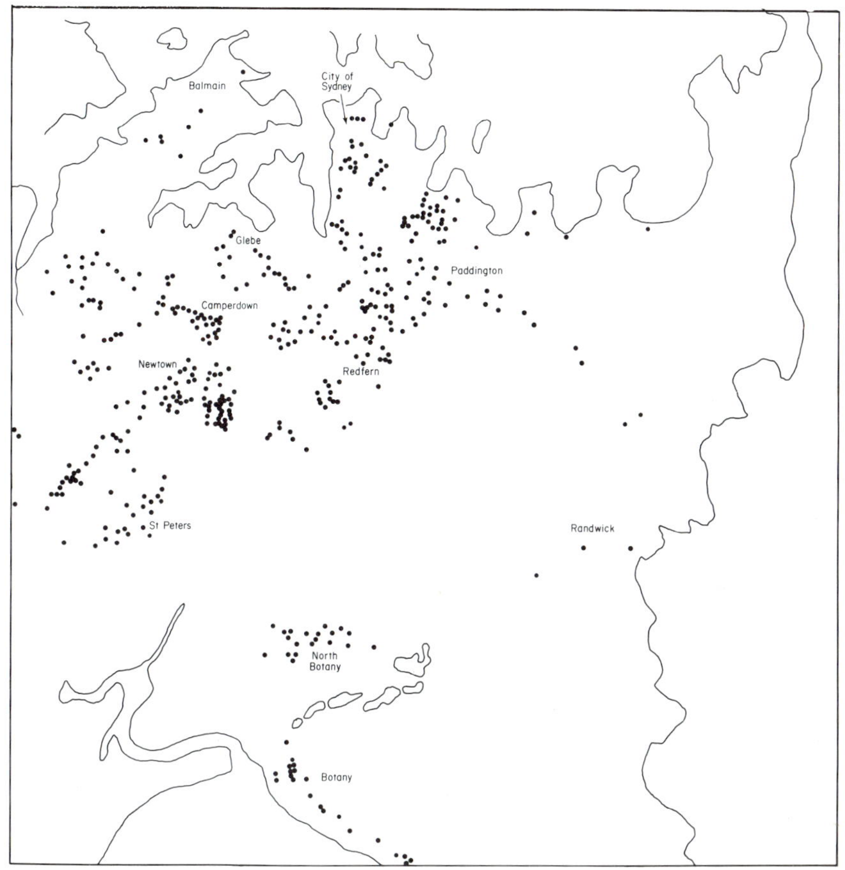

Figure 8 Distribution of typhoid cases, Sydney 1894

blame can be directed towards a series of less spectacular, more endemic diseases such as phthisis, diarrhoea, enteritis, convulsions, bronchitis and pneumonia, which extracted a heavy toll of life throughout the nineteenth century. When it comes to a broad overview of Sydney's mortality experience in these years there seems to be four distinctive periods:

1. *1788–1802*

The first few years of the new settlement were marked by very high and fluctuating death rates directly attributable to the arrival of convict ships and the transfer of ill and dying convicts to the land station. This, plus the privations of life associated with the unfamiliar environment, produced very high death rates. In 1790, for example, the crude death rate reached 90.5 per 1000 as a result of the high mortality following the arrival of the Second Fleet, and it reached 47 per 1000 in 1802 following the arrival of the convict vessels *Hercules, Atlas* and *Royal Admiral.*

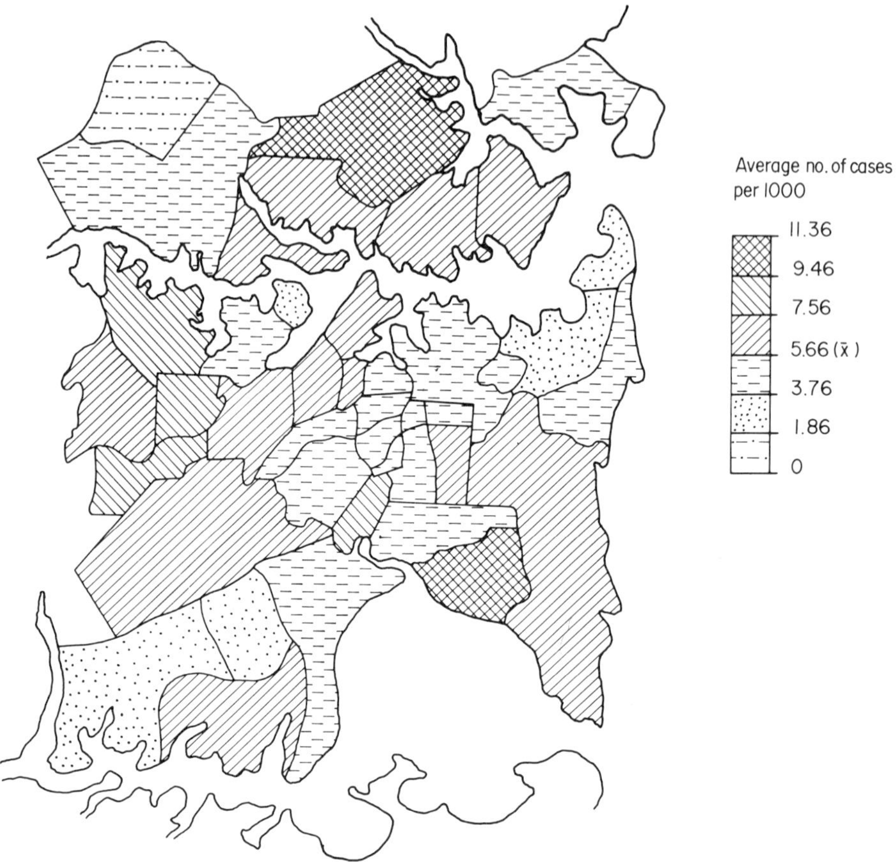

Figure 9 Average number of cases of infectious disease 1898–1900

2. *1803–25*

After 1802 Sydney entered a period of much lower mortality, largely brought about by improved conditions aboard many of the convict transports. The period was also notable, however, for the high levels of endemic disease and for the first appearance of epidemics of childhood infections.

3. *1826–42*

The sixteen years after 1825 were marked by steadily increasing mortality levels leading to the higher death rates of the period 1835–42. To a large extent this situation was brought about by the surge of free immigration in the late 1830s which transformed the town's demographic, social and epidemiological structure. As a consequence, epidemics of infectious disease became more frequent and more sustained. Influenza broke out in 1826 and 1838, whooping cough in 1828, measles in 1834–5 and scarlet fever in 1840–1. All produced a high death rate.

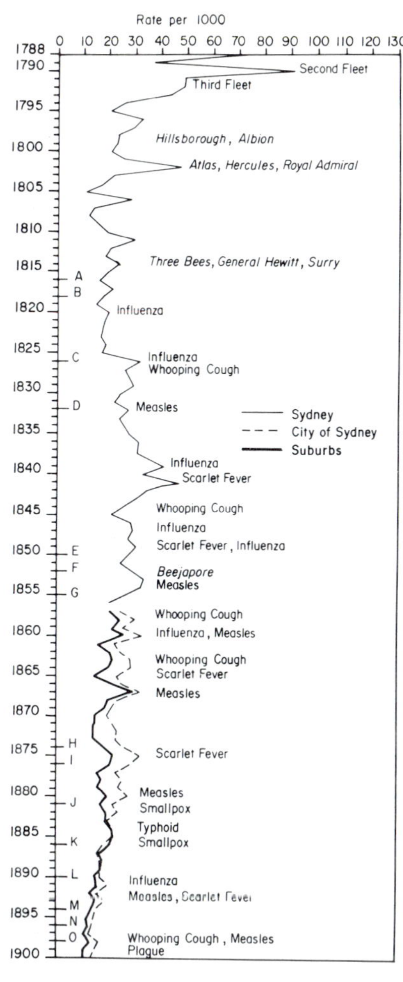

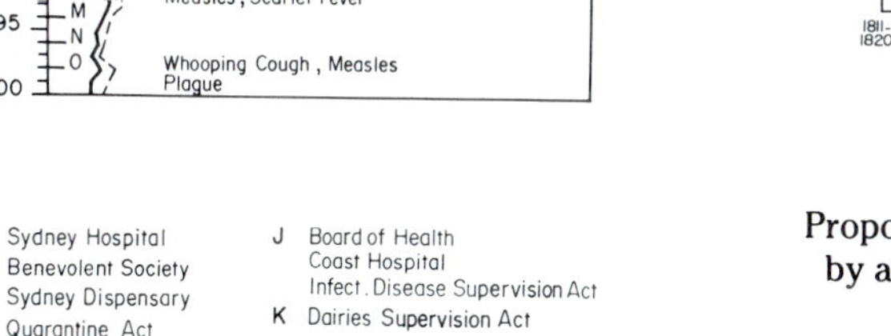

Figure 10
Sydney's death rate 1788–1900

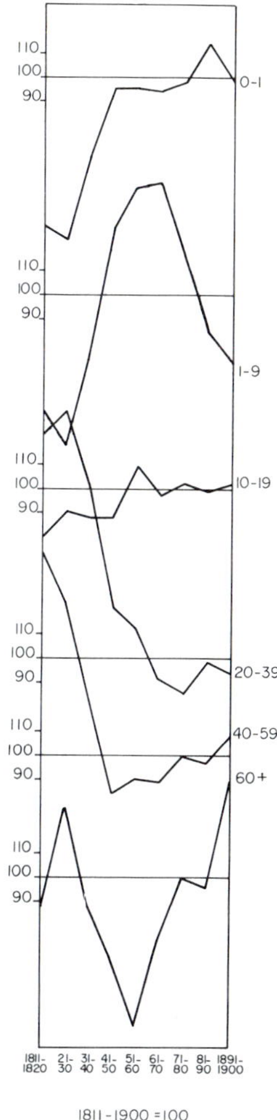

Figure 11
Proportion of total mortality by age groups 1811–1900

Curiously enough, the high mortality of this period seems to have occasioned little or no contemporary comment. Cumpston believes that this high mortality was produced by the dying-off of elderly convicts transported between 1788 and 1800 (Cumpston, 1931:593). Yet a close analysis of Sydney's burial registers for the years 1830–42 fails to reveal any noticeable increase in mortality at ages over 50 years. On the contrary, the contribution of this group to overall mortality declined in the decade 1831–40 when compared with the previous decade. The likely explanation for the increase in mortality during these years lies in the experience of the under five-year-old age group. Between 1835 and 1841 the number of deaths occurring in this age group increased more than fivefold and the overall contribution of this group to total mortality increased from less than one-quarter of all deaths in 1835–6 to almost 46 per cent by 1841.[5]

4. *1843–1900*
After 1843 Sydney experienced a fluctuating but generally declining death rate. From time to time the downward trend was temporarily arrested by short-lived peaks produced by epidemics of infectious disease. After 1876, however, such epidemics began to recede and the peaks of mortality they occasioned became lower and more spaced.

THE SELECTIVITY OF DEATH

In the years after 1788 death was highly selective in terms of those it struck down. Most at risk were convicts, the very young, the poor and the old. Males also seem to have been more at risk of premature deaths than females throughout most of the nineteenth century. To a large extent the limits of premature death were defined by the broad demographic and social parameters of Sydney's population. Consequently, prior to 1830 when the town's population was predominantly male adult-aged convicts, these groups were over-represented in Sydney's death registers. As the town's population changed in the 1830s so too did the demographic and social structure of death. The most important change came with the swing away from deaths being dominated by adult-aged males to a situation where infants and young children predominated. Table 3 and Figure 11 illustrate these broad changes by examining the proportion of total mortality by age group.[6] By the 1840s, infants aged under one year comprised almost 29 per cent of all deaths and this figure progressively increased over the following decades to reach more than 34 per cent by the 1880s. Young children (1–9 years) also experienced a rapid rise in importance although in their case the peak was reached during the 1860s before declining towards the end of the century. As the contribution of young children and infants increased, that of adults declined. From comprising almost 65 per cent of all deaths in the decade after 1811, the contribution of adults aged

5 An additional factor was probably the severe drought which affected the whole of southeastern Australia between February 1837 and December 1839.

6 Figure 11 illustrates these trends by the use of a divergency graph. For each age group the 100 line represents the contribution that the particular group made to total mortality between 1811 and 1900. Each decade is then plotted as an index number. Where the value lies above the 100 line it means that the particular age group made up a greater proportion of total mortality. This is merely expressing visually that, whereas infant deaths under one year made up 30.1 per cent of all deaths between 1811 and 1900, in the decade 1811–20 they contributed only 11.7 per cent.

Table 3 Age Distribution of Deaths 1811–1900 (%)

Age groups	*1811–20*	*1821–30*	*1831–40*	*1841–50*	*1851–60*	*1861–70*	*1871–80*	*1881–90*	*1891–1900*
0–1	11.71	9.94	20.75	28.92	29.00	28.58	29.79	34.55	29.75
1–9	9.57	7.07	13.68	23.63	27.00	30.84	25.48	15.96	13.51
10–19	2.78	3.16	3.06	3.07	3.80	3.38	3.56	3.45	3.54
20–39	34.21	35.86	30.51	21.54	20.04	16.18	15.12	17.53	16.65
40–59	30.71	26.70	20.20	13.90	14.80	14.54	16.24	15.78	17.69
60 +	11.64	17.26	11.79	8.93	5.21	9.86	13.36	12.73	18.85

Sources: Parish Registers; Convict Records, 1811–60; Registrar-General, Vital Statistics, 1860–1900.

Table 4 Age-Specific Mortality Rates, Sydney City and Suburbs, Selected Years 1841–1902 (number of deaths per 1000 population)

Age groups	*1841*	
	Males	*Females*
Under 2	247.9	253.6
2–7	72.3	57.1
7–14	24.2	25.6
14–20	14.8	22.0
21–44	29.6	24.7
45–60	70.9	37.6
60 +	193.8	179.2

Age groups	*1860–2*		*1870–2*		*1890–2*		*1900–2*	
	Males	*Females*	*Males*	*Females*	*Males*	*Females*	*Males*	*Females*
Under 1	182.2	157.4	149.1	151.1	178.3	148.7	143.7	125.5
1–9	22.6	23.5	16.1	15.6	9.9	9.1	5.7	5.9
10–19	3.6	3.3	3.3	2.7	3.0	2.3	2.7	1.9
20–29	10.5	7.1	8.3	5.6	6.3	5.3	5.0	4.4
30–39	14.5	11.1	12.4	11.1	9.6	8.6	8.1	7.0
40–49	17.5	15.6	18.0	18.0	16.1	12.1	13.7	9.5
50–59	26.9	22.4	24.9	23.3	26.2	18.8	23.1	15.6
60–69	45.7	47.4	50.3	45.0	49.9	33.9	45.7	35.1
70 +	119.4	120.3	105.0	123.4	110.0	100.3	107.3	96.0

Sources: 1841 — Parish Registers, Convict Records; 1860–1902 — Registrar-General, Vital Statistics and Census Records.

20–60 years rapidly fell away to only 30 per cent by the 1860s. The experience of the elderly (60+ years) reflects not only the early convict period but also the gradual increase in life expectancy and the ageing of the population which became important in the latter part of the century. From contributing less than 12 per cent of all deaths in 1811–20, the elderly's share increased to more than 17 per cent in 1821–30, declined to only 5 per cent in the middle of the century, and then progressively increased to almost 19 per cent by the 1890s.

Table 4 shows age-specific mortality rates for Sydney's male and female population for five periods between 1841 and 1902. The figures for 1841, although not comparable with later years because of the age categories used in the Census, nevertheless provide some evidence of the very high mortality rates prevailing in the early 1840s. The remainder of the table considers mortality rates by age for the period between 1860 and 1902. The most marked improvements over the 40 years after 1860 have related to the mortality experience of infants and children aged between one and nine years. Mortality rates for this age group were as high as 22.6 for males and 23.5 for females in 1860–2 and as low as 5.7 and 5.9 respectively 40 years later. By comparison, there was a much smaller improvement in the mortality of infants aged under one year. At most age groups the relative risk of mortality differed for males and females. Males, with only one or two exceptions, experienced higher mortality rates throughout the nineteenth century.

Figures 12 and 13 illustrate long-term trends in infant and child mortality by blending data from parish registers with data from official statistics. Figure 12 shows the annual death rate for children aged under five from 1810 to 1900.

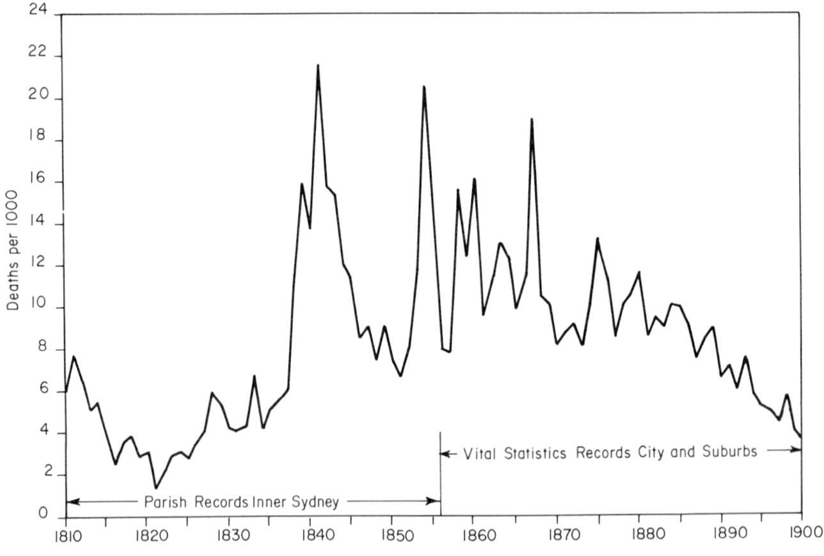

Figure 12 **Mortality rate of children under five years 1810–1900**

Immediately apparent is the rapid rise in the mortality rate in the late 1830s, coinciding with the increase in immigration and the growth in numbers of young children in Sydney. From a death rate of generally less than 6 per 1000 prior to 1838 mortality increased to more than 21 per 1000 in 1841, only to fall again to lower levels during the late 1840s. In the 25 years after 1850 the death rate for children under five generally fluctuated around high levels, although in epidemic years such as 1854 and 1867 young children could die at a rate in excess of 19–20 per 1000. After 1867, however, despite short-lived fluctuations, the mortality rate began a continuous decline until by the mid-1890s it had reached a figure of less than 6 per 1000.

With respect to infant mortality (i.e., deaths under one year per 1000 live births) (Figure 13), the period 1810–1900 saw wide and often spectacular swings in mortality. From a low figure of less than 90 deaths per 1000 live births before 1815, the rate fluctuated during the 1820s and 1830s before reaching a peak of 240 deaths per 1000 live births in 1838. After this, infant mortality declined rapidly until the 1850s when it peaked again, reaching a level of 254 deaths per 1000 live births in 1855. When official data became available in 1857 the city's infant mortality rate stood at 154.2. Thereafter it fluctuated wildly around a level of approximately 160 until towards the end of the century when it began to decline. By 1900 the infant mortality rate was 109.

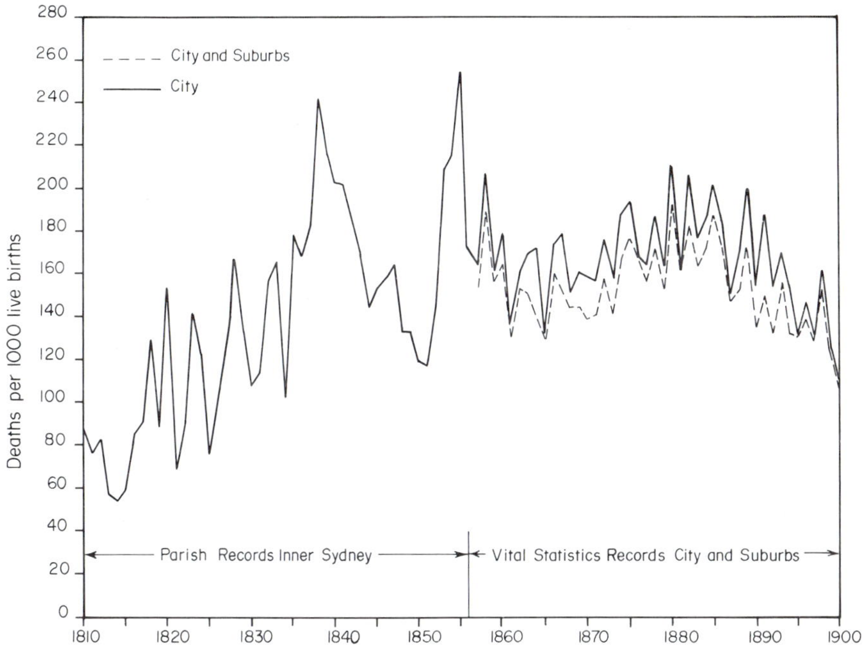

Figure 13 Infant mortality 1810–1900

THE CHANGING CAUSE OF DEATH

Regrettably there are few details as to the major causes of death during Sydney's first few decades. A series of fragmentary death returns for the General Hospital covering a series of years between 1803 and 1826 (Table 5) suggests a high level

Table 5 Major Cause of Death, General Hospital Sydney, Selected Years 1803–26

Cause of death	*1803*	*1811*	*1818*	*1826*
Dysentery	27	8	12	11
Diarrhoea/enteritis	—	—	8	3
Phthisis	4	—	8	8
Dropsy/hydrothorax	3	2	5	9
Accidents/violence	4	—	—	4
'Fever'	1	—	1	1
Venereal disease	1	2	1	2
Apoplexy	—	—	—	4
Debility	2	—	—	3
Scurvy	3	—	—	2
Other causes	—	6	10	17
Not stated	3	—	—	—
Total	48	18	45	64

Sources: *HRA* I, 4:517; Sydney Hospital, Quarterly Reports of Deaths.

Table 6 Major Cause of Death, Camperdown Cemetery Burials 1853–5

Cause of death	*Number*	*%*
'Natural'	686	23.8
Teething	224	7.8
Convulsions	153	5.3
Decline	142	4.9
Dysentery/diarrhoea	141	4.9
Consumption	136	4.7
Accidents/violence	100	3.5
Inflammation of lungs	98	3.4
Influenza/colds	93	3.2
Old age	88	3.1
Scarlet fever	80	2.8
Other gastrointestinal diseases	67	2.3
'Fever'	66	2.3
Heart disease	64	2.2
Dropsy	50	1.7
Other childhood infections[a]	46	1.6
Liver disease	43	1.5
Other	439	15.2
Not stated	161	5.6
Total	2877	100.0

Source: Camperdown Cemetery Burial Register, 1853–5.
[a] Whooping cough, croup, thrush, measles.

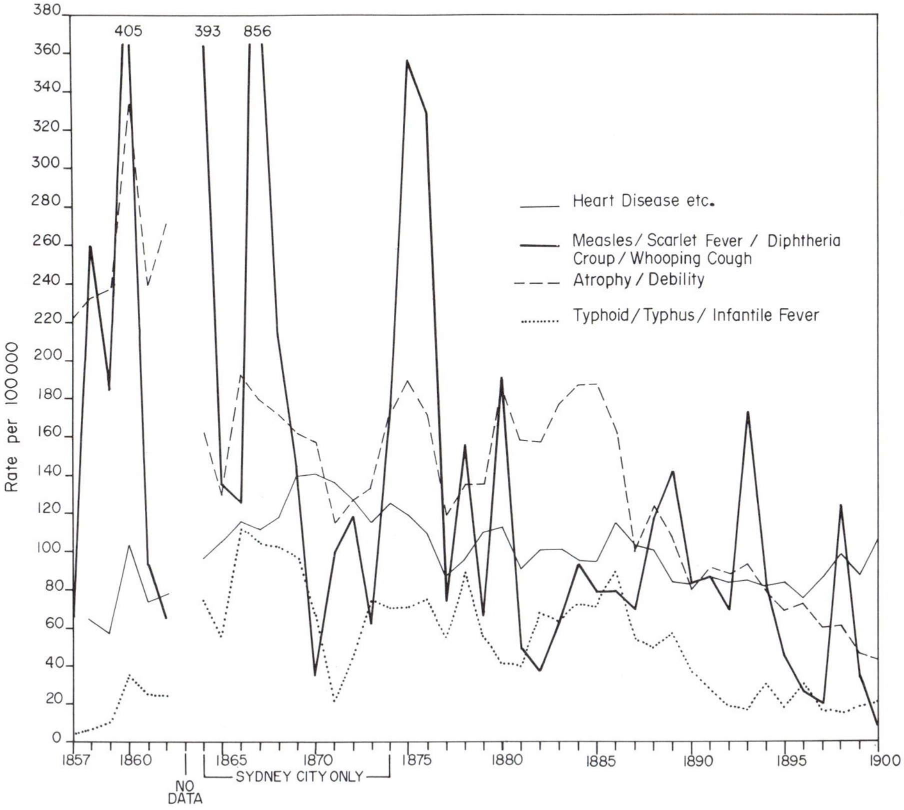
380
360
340
320
300
280
260
240
220
200
180
160
140
120
100
80
60
40
20
0
Rate per 100 000
405
393
856
Heart Disease etc.
Measles / Scarlet Fever / Diphtheria
Croup / Whooping Cough
Atrophy / Debility
Typhoid / Typhus / Infantile Fever
1857
1860
1865
1870
1875
1880
1885
1890
1895
1900
NO DATA
SYDNEY CITY ONLY

Figure 14 Mortality rates by cause 1857–1900

of deaths from dysentery (one-third of all deaths recorded), phthisis and dropsy. The first detailed material on cause of death in Sydney can be found in the Camperdown Cemetery burial registers in the early 1850s. Table 6 includes material extracted from this source for the years 1853–5. While the recognition of cause of death is far from ideal (particularly in so far as 24 per cent of all deaths were recorded as being from 'natural' causes) this table does provide some information on the major causes of death in the early 1850s.

After 1857 the Registrar-General's official returns regularly recorded cause of death in Sydney and this source forms the basis of Figures 14 and 15 which record mortality rates per 100 000 by cause for the period 1857–1900. Figure 14 illustrates the downward trend after 1857 in the mortality rate from the major childhood infections. Rather than a continuous decline, what is significant is that the high peaks of mortality associated with epidemics became less spectacular and more spaced. The regular periodicity developed by particular childhood infections can be seen in Figure 16 which records the total number of deaths for Sydney in the period 1856–1900. By the 1890s the death rate from childhood infections had

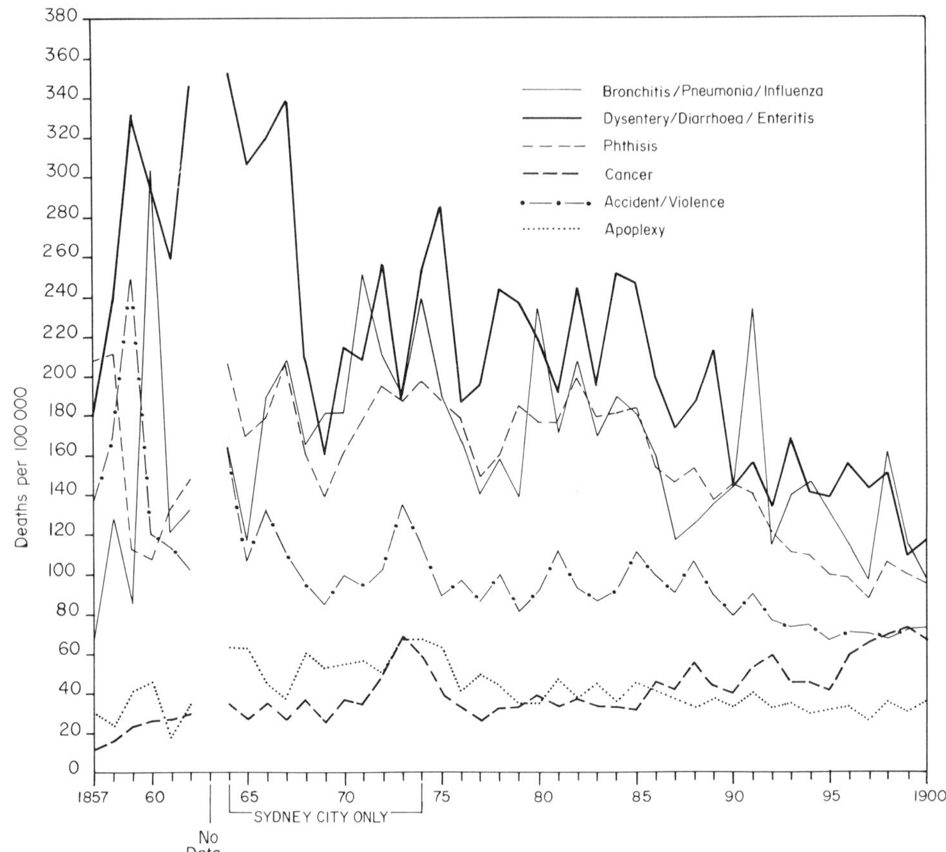

Figure 15 **Mortality rates by cause 1857–1900**

fallen to below 100 with the exception of the epidemic years of 1893 and 1898, and by 1900 the rate was below 20 deaths per 100 000. The major enteric diseases (dysentery, diarrhoea, enteritis) have played an important role as a leading cause of death throughout most of Sydney's early history. Deaths from this cause were at their highest in the late 1850s to early 1860s and in the period 1870–85. After 1885 their importance declined until by 1900 the death rate from this cause stood at 120 per 100 000. This decline probably took place first in deaths from dysentery and then diarrhoea and enteritis. Even by 1900 these three diseases were the leading cause of death in Sydney. Deaths from atrophy and debility also show evidence of a decline after 1885. By the end of the century mortality from these causes was only one-quarter of what it had been fifteen years before. Mortality from bronchitis/pneumonia and influenza was strongly influenced by the influenza epidemics of 1860 and 1891 but generally remained at a high level from 1860 until 1886.

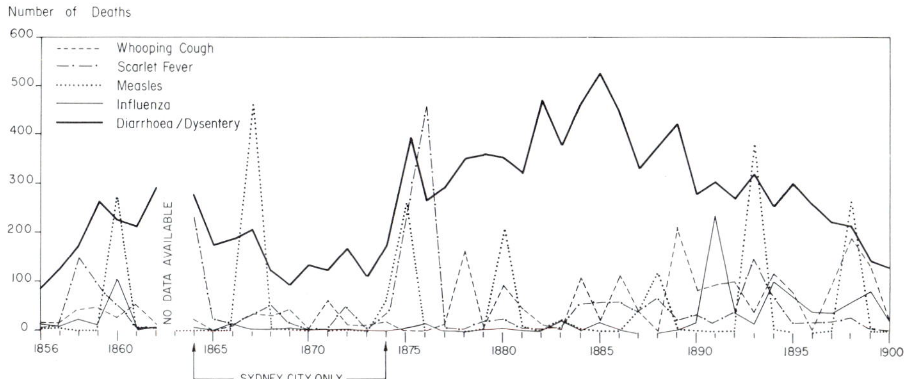

Figure 16 Number of deaths from major infections 1857–1900

Changes in the top ten leading causes of death provide another way of evaluating the change in major cause of death. Referred to here as the 'leading cause of death' they are ranked in order of importance with respect to their contribution to total deaths. Four periods between 1858 and 1900 have been chosen for illustration (Table 7). In 1858–9 six of the top ten leading causes of death were childhood diseases and the top three were all diseases of the first four years of life. Only accidents and violence, phthisis, and lung and brain disease intruded into the list. Sixteen years later infectious disease accounted for seven of the top ten causes of death, with scarlet fever and phthisis topping the list followed by a number of childhood diseases. By the early 1880s infectious disease still held pride of place although by now phthisis had consolidated its position and was the city's leading cause of death. It was a place that it was to occupy for at least the next 25 years. Although childhood infections still figured prominently after 1880, other diseases as much associated with the aged as the young, such as bronchitis, pneumonia, cancer and heart disease, began to play a more important role. By the end of the century heart disease and cancer were among the top five causes of death.

When the examination of cause of death is made more age-specific what is striking is how little the major cause of death changed for some age groups over the latter part of last century (Tables 8–10). For infants aged under one year, for example, the major causes of death altered very little between 1850 and 1900. Diarrhoea, enteritis, convulsions and atrophy/debility remained the principal causes of infant death for these 50 years. Much the same applies to young and middle-aged adults. For both groups, phthisis, accidents and violence, heart disease and pneumonia claimed most victims. For Sydney's elderly population the major causes of death seem to have been established very early in the city's development and changed only minimally over the last half of the century. 'Old age', heart disease, cancer, apoplexy and bronchitis consistently claimed most lives in this age group throughout the last 50 years of the nineteenth century.

Table 7 Ten Leading Causes of Death, Sydney and Suburbs, 1858–9, 1875–6, 1882–3, 1899–1900

Rank	*Cause*	*% of deaths*	*Rank*	*Cause*	*% of deaths*
	1858–9			1875–6	
1	Convulsions	9.9	1	Scarlet fever	7.9
2	Atrophy/debility	9.1	2	Phthisis	7.2
3	Teething	7.4	3	Atrophy/debility	7.1
4	Accidents	6.5	4	Diarrhoea	7.0
5	Diarrhoea	5.5	5	Convulsions	4.5
6	Phthisis	5.5	6	Bronchitis	4.3
7	Scarlet fever	5.1	7	Accidents/violence	3.6
8	Dysentery	4.1	8	Pneumonia	3.5
9	Lung disease	3.3	9	Measles	3.1
10	Brain disease	3.1	10	Typhoid	2.9
	1882–3			1899–1900	
1	Phthisis	9.8	1	Phthisis	8.6
2	Atrophy/debility	8.6	2	Heart disease	8.5
3	Diarrhoea	8.1	3	Enteritis	8.4
4	Bronchitis	5.3	4	Accidents/violence	6.4
5	Convulsions	5.2	5	Cancer	6.2
6	Heart disease	5.1	6	Pneumonia	5.2
7	Accidents/violence	4.6	7	Atrophy/debility	3.9
8	Pneumonia	4.2	8	Premature birth	3.6
9	Typhoid	3.4	9	Bronchitis	3.2
10	Gastritis/enteritis	2.8	10	Bright's disease	3.0

Source: Registrar-General, Vital Statistics, 1858–1900.

Table 8 Principal Cause of Death by Age Group 1850–1

Cause	*% of deaths*	*Cause*	*% of deaths*
0–1		1–9	
'Natural'	21.6	Scarlet fever	19.5
Convulsions	14.6	Teething	15.8
Diarrhoea	13.4	'Natural'	10.5
Teething	12.7	'Fever'	6.8
Dysentery	10.8	Convulsions	5.3
10–19		20–39	
'Fever'	20.0	Phthisis	15.2
Decline	16.0	Accidents/violence	13.6
Accidents/violence	16.0	'Natural'	9.6
Phthisis	8.0	Heart Disease	7.9
		Dysentery	6.2
40–59		60 +	
'Natural'	23.6	Old age	56.8
Phthisis	9.0	'Natural'	7.6
Dysentery	7.0	Diarrhoea	4.2
Accidents/violence	6.0	Apoplexy	4.2
Liver disease	6.0	Dropsy	4.2
Heart disease	6.0	Bronchitis	4.2

Source: Camperdown Cemetery Burial Register, 1850–1.

Table 9 Principal Cause of Death by Age Group 1882–3

Cause	*% of deaths*	*Cause*	*% of deaths*
0–1		1–9	
Atrophy/debility	21.9	Diarrhoea	11.4
Diarrhoea	15.5	Convulsions	7.8
Convulsions	11.4	Bronchitis	6.9
Premature birth	7.3	Croup	6.6
Bronchitis	6.8	Pneumonia	6.1
Gastritis/enteritis	6.7	Cephalitis	5.7
10–19		20–39	
Phthisis	21.7	Phthisis	31.3
Typhus	16.8	Accidents/violence	9.6
Accidents/violence	9.9	Typhus	9.0
Heart disease	7.5	Heart disease	6.2
Pneumonia	5.1	Pneumonia	5.5
Cephalitis	4.0		
40–59		60+	
Phthisis	18.3	Old age	24.6
Heart disease	9.1	Heart disease	10.6
Pneumonia	6.7	Bronchitis	9.6
Accidents/violence	6.2	Apoplexy	6.0
Cancer	4.8	Cancer	4.6

Source: Registrar-General, Vital Statistics, 1882–3.

Table 10 Principal Cause of Death by Age Group 1899–1900

Cause	*% of deaths*	*Cause*	*% of deaths*
0–1		1–9	
Enteritis	23.2	Enteritis	11.8
Atrophy/debility	14.3	Pneumonia	11.8
Premature birth	14.2	Whooping cough	6.7
Diarrhoea	6.0	Accidents/violence	6.2
Convulsions	6.0	Tubercular meningitis	6.1
Pneumonia	4.3	Inflammation of brain	6.0
10–19		20–39	
Accidents/violence	16.8	Phthisis	25.0
Phthisis	12.1	Accidents/violence	9.5
Typhoid	11.2	Heart disease	6.8
Heart disease	9.6	Pneumonia	4.7
Plague	5.8	Typhoid	4.2
40–59		60+	
Phthisis	14.2	Old age	13.8
Heart disease	14.2	Heart disease	12.4
Cancer	13.3	Cancer	11.3
Accidents/violence	8.3	Apoplexy	6.9
Bright's disease	6.0	Bronchitis	6.0
Pneumonia	4.6	Bright's disease	4.9

Source: Registrar-General, Vital Statistics, 1899–1900.

MORTALITY DECLINE IN THE LATE NINETEENTH CENTURY

Towards the end of the nineteenth century the incidence and mortality fell for a wide range of infectious diseases for which no effective medical treatment existed. Deaths from phthisis commenced a rapid and continuous decline after 1885, long before the introduction of any specific therapy. Mortality from diphtheria declined rapidly after 1889, some years before the introduction of a specific antitoxin (March 1895) or before the specialized diphtheria ward was opened at Sydney Hospital and tracheotomies became more widely performed (July 1893). Many other infectious diseases such as scarlet fever, measles and the enteric diseases followed suit in the period 1885–93 (Figure 17). In some cases general improvements in the quality and supply of water and milk products and the disposal of sewage may have influenced the decline. Improvements in the purity of the milk supply and general surveillance of dairies that followed the passing of the Dairies Supervision

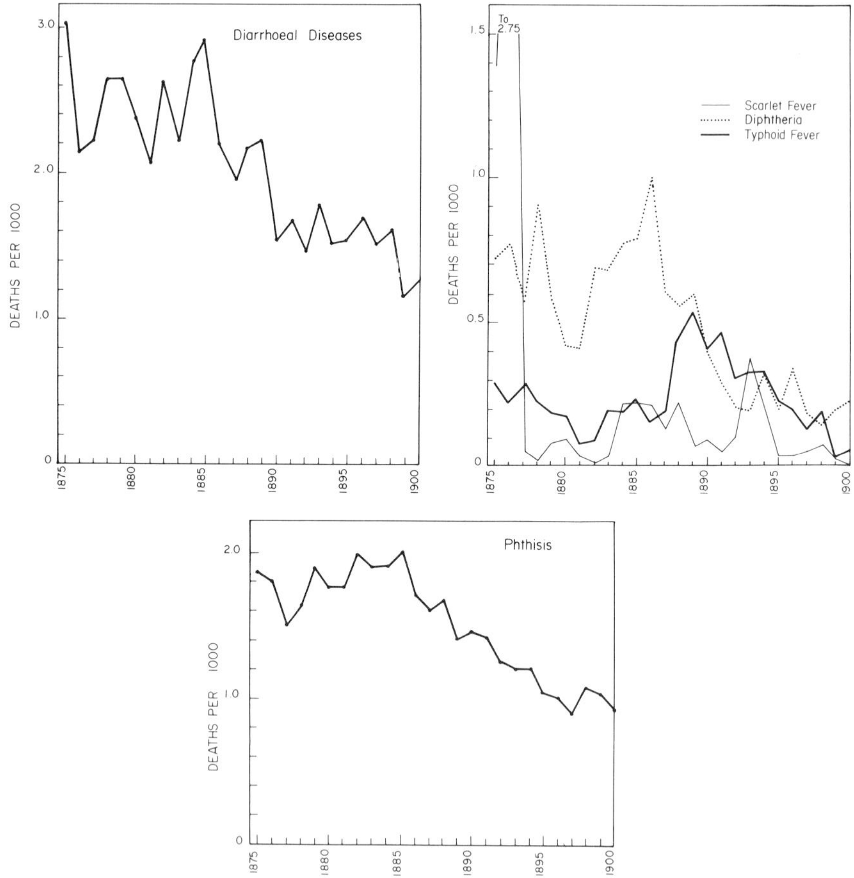

Figure 17 Death rate from selected diseases 1875–1900

Act of 1886 contributed to the decline in infant deaths from a variety of causes such as tabes mesenterica, scrofula, and diarrhoea (see Lewis, 1980: 193–207). In the 1880s to early 1890s fresh water mains were extended to a large number of suburbs such as Balmain, Leichhardt, Randwick and Marrickville, and in 1887 the Board of Water Supply and Sewage commenced operation and a new sewage outfall at Bondi came into use the same year. Certainly all this would seem to have contributed to the decline in deaths from typhoid, dysentery and diarrhoea. Yet even by 1900 the majority of households in Sydney were still dependent upon primitive means of sewage disposal and were the recipients of less than pure water and unadulterated food. It is also highly doubtful as to whether there was any noticeable improvement in diet and/or living conditions during the last two decades of the nineteenth century. On the contrary, it would seem that housing standards and living conditions in Sydney actually declined during the period 1880–1900 despite broad improvements in public health. It thus remains a mystery as to why many infectious diseases began to decline in virulence at just that moment when there was a rapid surge in immigration and urbanization, a period of economic depression, a general increase in urban population densities, an increase in household size and a general deterioration in working and living conditions. It is possible that the geographical shift in population away from the City of Sydney to suburban areas which became important in the 1880s contributed in some way to improving health. Yet living and working conditions in many of the newly emerging inner suburbs such as Waterloo, Alexandria, St Peters, Botany, Enfield and Balmain were in many ways as marginal and depressed as those in the central city. Perhaps the answer lies in the interplay of two factors: (1) the changing demographic structure of the population, and (2) the possibility that the decline was brought about by some basic change in the character and make-up of the diseases themselves. After 1885 Sydney like many western urban areas had experienced a marked fall in fertility levels, an ageing of the population and a change in the completed family size/number of children born to married women. Quite possibly, as Gandevia points out, these developments influenced the course and virulence of a number of childhood infections, particularly for those diseases where mortality was most severe during the first two years of life (e.g. whooping cough, measles, scarlet fever, diphtheria). In such cases the possibility of high mortality may have been substantially reduced by the absence of an older child from the household (Gandevia, 1978:132). It is also possible that many of the diseases in question underwent a change in infectivity and virulence during the latter part of the nineteenth century.

SEASONAL RHYTHM OF MORTALITY

It would seem that a particular seasonal rhythm of mortality has been a feature of Sydney's demographic scene at least from the beginning of the nineteenth century. By the first decade of the 1800s the pattern was well established and largely consisted of a summer high (November–February) and a winter low (June–October). Before 1811 this seasonal pattern was complicated by the surge of deaths that inevitably followed the arrival of particular convict transports such

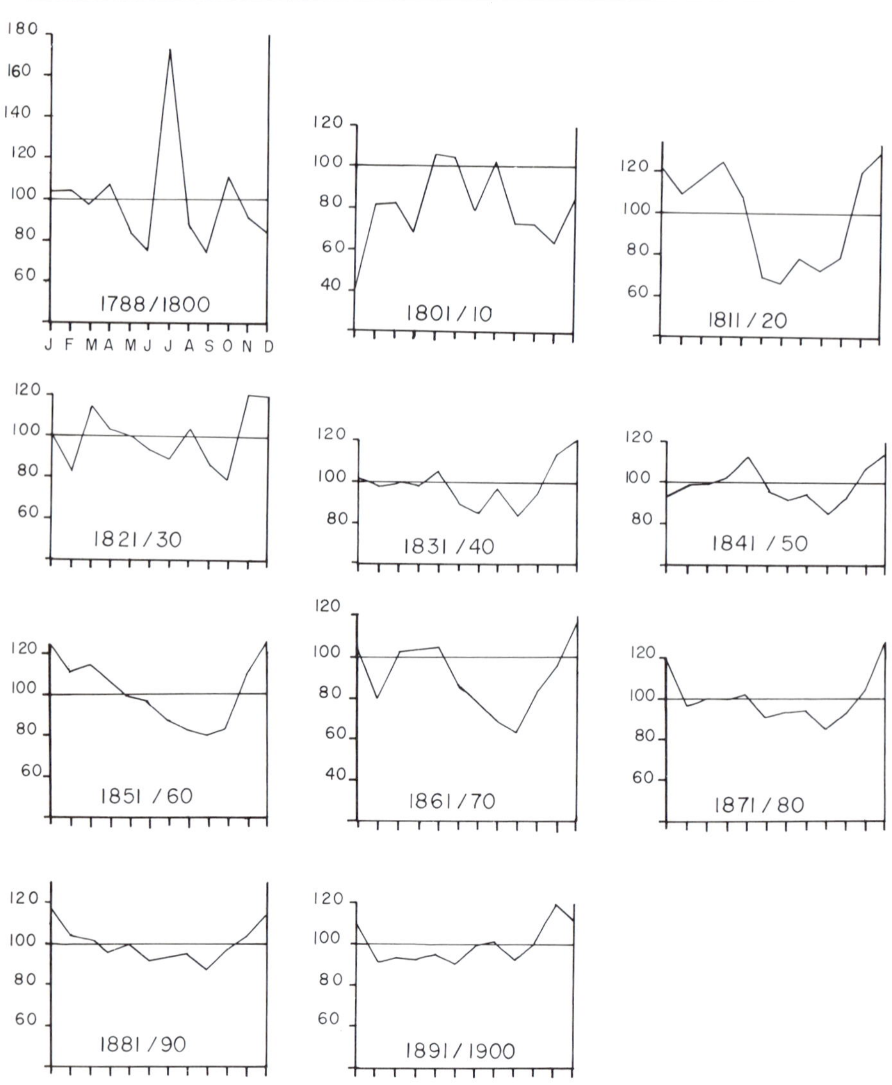

Figure 18 Monthly mortality rate 1788–1900

as in 1790 (responsible for the July peak 1788–1800 on Figure 18).[7] Particular epidemics could also produce temporary disruptions to the summer high/winter low regime. The measles epidemic of March/April 1854, for instance, was partly

[7] Figure 18 is calculated on the basis of a monthly death index where the index for a particular month represents

$$1200 \times \frac{\text{number of deaths in the particular month}}{\text{total number of deaths in the year}}$$

(See Momiyama and Katayama, 1966.)

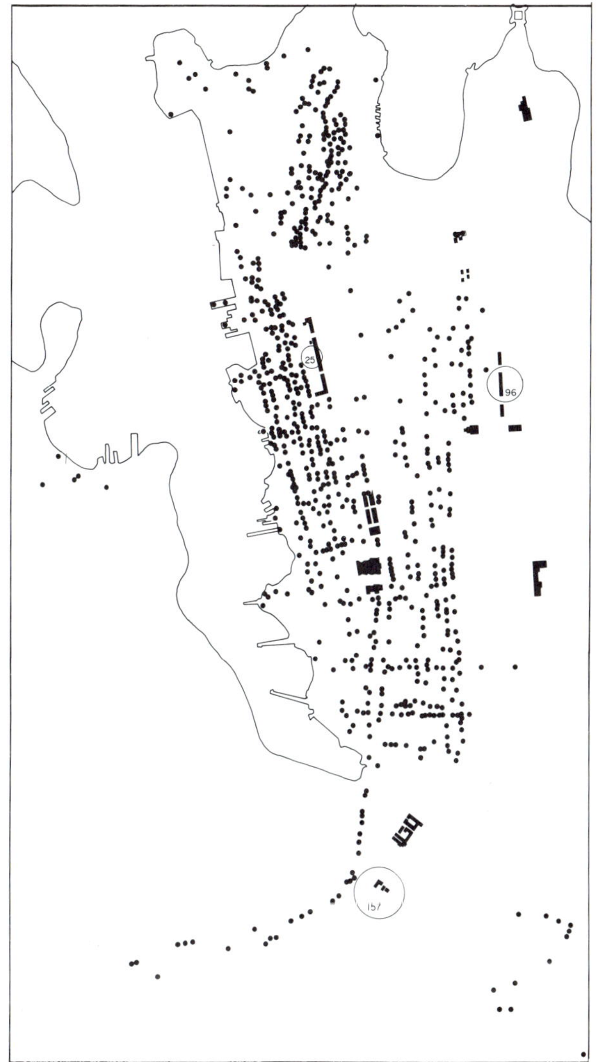

Figure 19 Distribution of deaths, inner Sydney 1841

responsible for the extension of the summer peak from January to April 1851–60 while the severe outbreak of measles in 1867 helps explain the high peak in the period March–May 1861–70. The summer peak in mortality seems attributable to the increased incidence of gastrointestinal diseases such as dysentery, diarrhoea and enteritis as well as typhoid fever. The magnitude of this seasonal pattern of death changed little during the nineteenth century and it was not until after 1900 that improved hygiene and food preservation techniques helped to lower the number of deaths from enteric diseases so that the prevalence of winter respiratory diseases, particularly influenza and pneumonia, became more important.

SPATIAL PATTERNS

Throughout most of the nineteenth century substantial variations existed in the spatial pattern of mortality within Sydney. To a large extent such patterns reflected the spatial distribution of Sydney's social classes as well as a variety of other factors such as the location of noxious industry, poorly drained land and swamps. Concentrations of high mortality were, therefore, closely related to depressed and crowded living and working conditions, poor sanitation, polluted water supplies, contaminated food and marginal nutritional levels. All these factors led to a higher

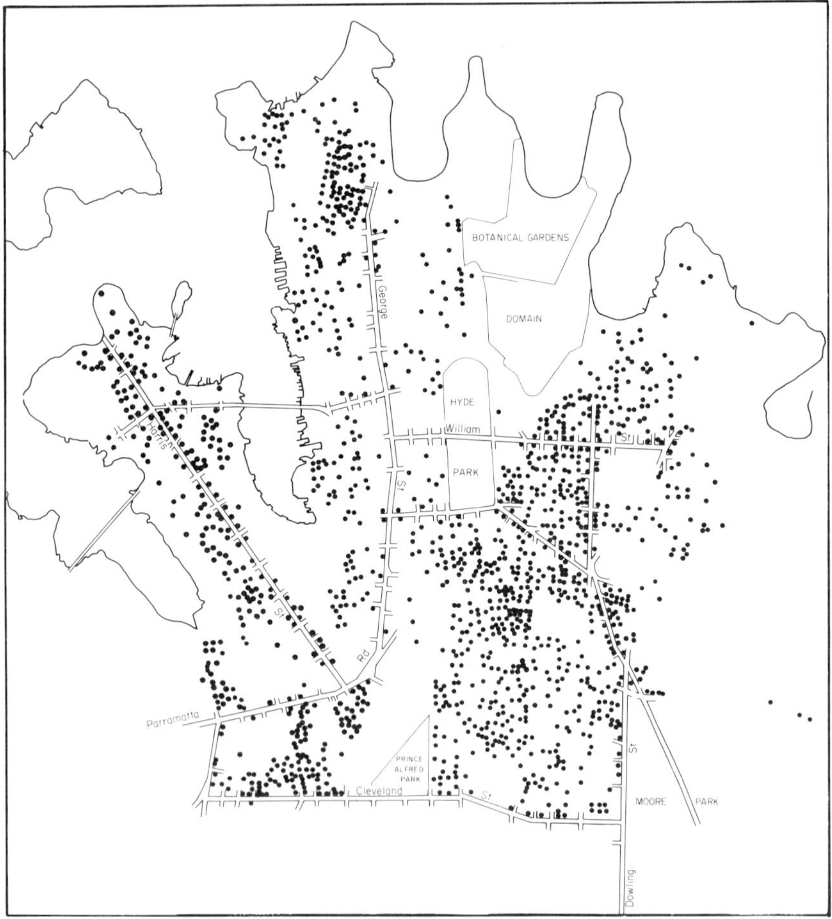

Figure 20 Distribution of deaths, City of Sydney 1889

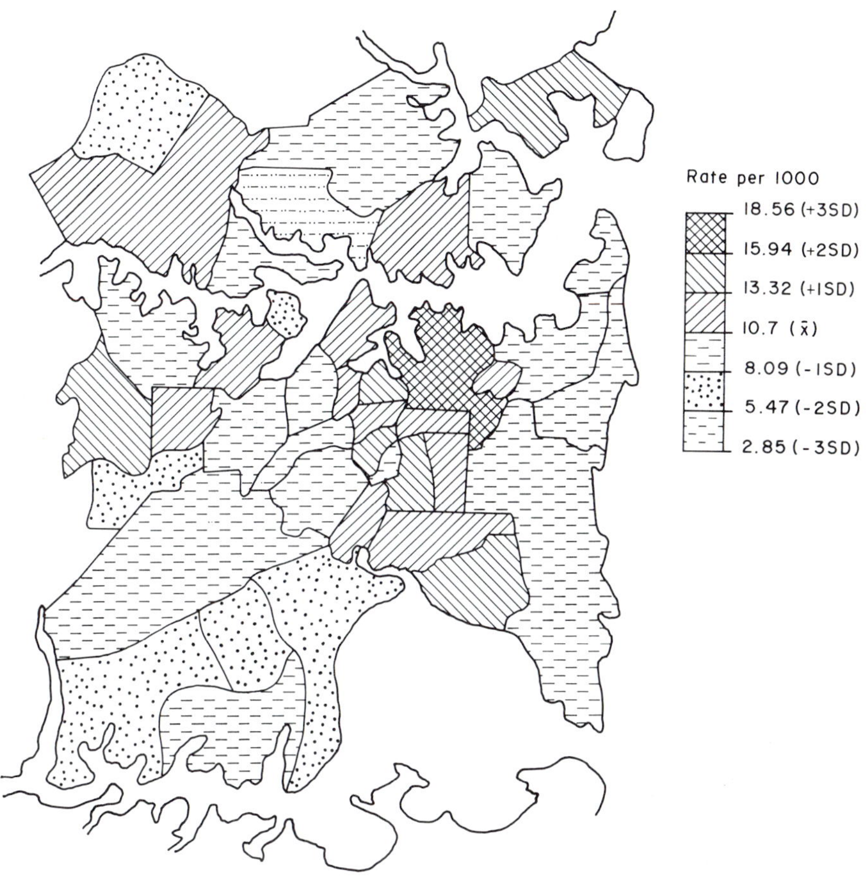

Figure 21 Crude death rate, Sydney 1900

incidence of disease, particularly infectious disease, as well as accidents. The only complication to such a pattern was where a particular institution existed to cater for the sick, elderly or destitute (such as the Benevolent Asylum) or where a particular suburb supported a higher proportion of elderly people. Towards the last quarter of the century this last factor, that is, the distribution of elderly population, came to play almost as important a role in explaining the spatial distribution of mortality as did the distribution of the city's poor.

Within the City of Sydney the distribution of deaths in 1841 illustrated many of the above points (Figure 19). Deaths were overly concentrated in areas of working-class residence, particularly in the lower Rocks, the area west of George Street fringing Darling Harbour and the area to the immediate east and south of the Town Hall. Apart from these spatial concentrations, 157 deaths occurred at the Benevolent Asylum, 96 at the Hospital and 25 at the Barracks. By 1889 the spatial pattern of death still showed some similarity to that of 1841 (Figure 20). The lower

Rocks area retained its importance as a zone of high mortality, as did the residential area fringing Darling Harbour. The major concentration of deaths in 1889, however, reflected the shift in working-class population that had taken place in preceding years to the residential areas east and south of Hyde Park at Woolloomooloo and Surry Hills. Finally, the growth of working-class residential areas in Pyrmont, Ultimo and Chippendale accounts for the concentration of deaths in these areas. By the turn of the century, although Sydney's death rate had fallen below 12 per 1000, important spatial variations remained, reflecting basic social and economic distinctions. In 1900 the death rate per 1000 varied across Sydney from a high 16.6 in the City of Sydney to a low 4.4 in Lane Cove (Figure 21). Broadly a concentric pattern of high central values–low suburban values emerges but the pattern, like earlier years, was complicated by a number of factors. In the first place, it remained true that the higher the social class of a suburb the lower its mortality rate. Thus, areas like Vaucluse and Hunters Hill had rates well below the average. In the second place, newly settled residential areas such as Drummoyne and Marsfield also had low mortality rates. Thirdly, suburbs that had a more elderly population structure or that supported institutions for the care of the aged, ill or destitute generally had a higher mortality rate. Overall, however, the suburbs with the highest mortality were those inner-city areas where blue-collar or unskilled workers resided and/or where noxious industry had located.

CHAPTER THREE

'All Dead! All Dead!'

The Great Sickness of 1789

ONE OF THE MOST intriguing and unresolved episodes in Australia's early history concerns the year 1789 when from all accounts a severe epidemic of an unknown infectious disease ravaged the Aboriginal population in the vicinity of Sydney. Very little information has survived concerning this disaster save a handful of contemporary accounts long mulled over by scholars. What these accounts suggest is that the Aboriginal population living between Botany Bay and Broken Bay were visited by a virulent epidemic disease sometime during March or April 1789 which caused great mortality and socio-economic disruption and for some inexplicable reason left the immigrant white population almost completely untouched. What disease was it that caused such havoc? Where did it come from? Why were no Europeans affected? Was the epidemic as severe and as widespread as the contemporaries believed? These questions remain unresolved to this day. Was the disease really smallpox as most contemporaries and later writers came to believe or was it some more common infectious disease introduced as a completely new infection into a totally non-immune population where it adopted a particularly virulent and unfamiliar nature? Whether smallpox or not, the contemporary accounts were unanimous in assessing the effects of the epidemic. It appeared almost overnight as if from nowhere and in a very short time devastated the Aboriginal population in the Sydney region. Possibly thousands of Aboriginals were swept away by it in a few months and if this were true then the epidemic represents the greatest single disaster suffered by Australia's Aboriginal population.

The 1789 epidemic thus provides a fascinating epidemiological puzzle. Not only was it Sydney's first major epidemic but it was also the greatest mortality crisis to affect the Sydney area. Regrettably, it is also the epidemic to leave the faintest trace in the historical record. Unlike the later epidemics to be examined in this book, the 1789 outbreak has left us no hard data with which to reconstruct the origin, impact and effects of a major mortality disaster. In addition, the written record consists mainly of the passing comments of contemporary observers who generally provide insufficiently detailed descriptions to allow us to pass judgement on the origin, nature and course of the disease. In consequence any attempt to reconstruct this earliest of epidemics must battle with a lack of detailed information, with ambiguity, contradiction and partisan comment, and must rely heavily upon the accounts of contemporary observers. The situation is further complicated by some of the later medical writers who have been somewhat too free in the inferences they have drawn from the early accounts. Yet many questions surrounding this epidemic deserve answers. Was it smallpox? What was the source of the infection? What was the mortality rate? Was it as severe a crisis as the contemporaries have led us to believe? Why did the European population escape unscathed? What was the spatial extent of the epidemic and its manner of diffusion? Given the nature of the evidence, it seems inevitable that our answers be somewhat speculative but there seem little doubt that some of the original material has been subjected to misinterpretation and that a careful reassessment is long overdue.

EVIDENCE OF A MAJOR EPIDEMIC

Evidence of an extensive epidemic breaking out in the Sydney area in April 1789 derives from the accounts of many of the contemporary observers of Sydney's first few years, such as Collins, Tench, Scott, Phillip, Bradley and King. All are clear in their reference to a major epidemic and were awed by its extent and spectacular mortality. As Collins wrote,

> Early in the month [April], and throughout its continuance, the people whose business called them down the Harbour daily reported, that they found, either in excavations of the rock, or lying upon the beaches and points of the different coves . . . the bodies of many of the wretched natives of this country. (Collins, 1971:65)

Somewhat earlier Sergeant James Scott had recorded in his diary that while on a routine work party to cut timber near Sydney he 'found three nativs under a rock, vis, a man and two Boys (of which one Boy was dead). The Govorner being Acquented with it, ordered the Man and Boy to the Hospital under Care of the Surgion the having the Small pox' (quoted in Cobley, 1963:26).

The epidemic seems to have extended up the harbour in all directions and as Tench states:

> An extraordinary calamity was now observed among the natives. Repeated accounts brought by our boats of finding bodies of the Indians in all the coves and inlets of the harbour . . . (Tench, 1979:146)

When assessing the diseases common to the native population around Sydney, Collins summed up the epidemic in the following terms:

> In the year 1789 they were visited by a disorder which raged among them with all the appearance and virulence of the Small-pox. The number that it swept off, by their own accounts, was incredible. At that time a native was living with us; and on taking him down to the harbour to look for his former companions, those who witnessed his expression and

agony can never forget either. He looked anxiously around him in the different coves we visited; not a vestige on the sand was to be found of human foot; the excavations in the rocks were filled with the putrid bodies of those who had fallen victims to the disorder; not a living person was any where to be met with. It seemed as if, flying from the contagion, they had left the dead to bury the dead. He lifted up his hands and eyes in silent agony for some time; at last he exclaimed, 'All dead! All dead!' . . . As proof of the numbers of those miserable people who were carried off by this disorder, Bennillong told us, that his friend Cole-be's tribe being reduced by its effects to three persons. (Collins, 1971:597–8)

Finally, Bradley records his impressions of sailing into Port Jackson on his return from the Cape of Good Hope:

From the great number of dead Natives found in every part of the Harbour, it appears that the small-pox had made dreadful havock among them. We did not see a Canoe or a Native the whole way coming up the Harbour, and were told that scarce any had been seen lately, except laying dead in and about their miserable habitations. (quoted in Cobley, 1963:35)

WHICH POX?

When it comes to deciding what disease was responsible for this great mortality later medical writers and historians have accepted the views put forward by the contemporaries such as Collins, Tench and Phillip. Although there seems to have been some initial doubt as to what agent was responsible for the epidemic, such uncertainty seems to have disappeared when a family suffering from the disease was brought into the settlement and closely examined.

The symptoms and general appearance of these cases seem to have struck a familiar chord and Collins wrote:

that it was the Small-pox there was scarcely a doubt, for the person seized by it was affected exactly as Europeans are who have that disorder and on many that had recovered from it we saw the traces, in some the ravages on the face. (Collins, 1971:598)

Tench seems almost as convinced when he wrote,

pustules similar to those occasioned by the smallpox, were thickly spread on the bodies . . . eruptions covered the poor boy from head to foot. (Tench, 1979:146)

Finally, Phillip in his detailed report on the settlement to Lord Sydney speculates on the origin of the outbreak and categorically states the disease to have been smallpox (Cobley, 1963:141).

Unfortunately no account provides us with a sufficiently detailed description of the disease so as to prove conclusively that it was smallpox. The contemporaries and later writers seem to have been swayed by the appearance of eruptions, fever and facial scarring. This evidence remains at best inconclusive. Smallpox was often misdiagnosed before the early twentieth century and it was often very difficult to distinguish a mild case from that of chickenpox (varicella). Chickenpox was not fully differentiated from smallpox until the end of the nineteenth century and it is thus quite possible that the infection that broke out in 1789 was not smallpox at all but chickenpox introduced into a population with no previous acquaintance with the disease. As such the resulting infection would probably have been very different from the chickenpox that English doctors were familiar with back home. Normally chickenpox is a benign but highly contagious disease of childhood, but when transported to a different climatic and health environment and let loose upon a previously unexposed and non-immune population it could become an extremely severe disease. It is also possible that serious and lethal complications could develop. The intense itching of the disease tempts scratching and given the hot moist climate and lack of personal hygiene this could easily have led to suppurative bacterial infection and permanent scarring particularly on the face. The symptoms of chickenpox also closely resemble those of smallpox. The disease begins with a fever followed within a few days by the sudden eruption of crops of skin lesions. Headache, backache, shivering, a sore throat and cough are normal occurrences for both diseases in adults. Difficulty in swallowing and a craving for fluids are also common. Tench's description of the man brought into the settlement who suffered from shivering fits, craved water and frequently pointed to his throat which in its obstructed and tender state restricted gargling (Tench, 1979:147) could as easily describe the symptoms of chickenpox as smallpox. In the case of chickenpox the rash is largely centripetal, being heaviest on the trunk, particularly in the hollow of the small of the back and between the shoulder blades, as well as on arms and thighs. In the case of smallpox the eruptions are, by contrast, largely centrifugal, that is, on the face, legs and forearms.[1] Unfortunately the contemporary descriptions of those suffering from the disease are not clinically detailed enough to reveal which disease was actually involved, although Tench's description of the cases brought into the town with eruptions 'thickly spread on the bodies' and of the boy being 'covered from head to foot' suggest a more widespread rash than is usual with smallpox.

In the end, whether the disease was smallpox or chickenpox remains debatable. The later authorities such as Cumpston and Tidswell have been swayed by the accounts of Collins, Tench and Phillip but the evidence could equally point to chickenpox being responsible for the outbreak.

THE ORIGIN OF THE EPIDEMIC

One of the most intriguing features of the epidemic concerns the source of the infection. The actual origin of the infection remains shrouded in obscurity despite a great deal of speculation at the time of the outbreak and subsequently. As far as can be ascertained there is no record of either smallpox or chickenpox cases in the settlement prior to 1789. In addition, after the arrival of the First Fleet in 1788 there were no shipping arrivals, apart from storeships plying to and from Norfolk Island, until the arrival of the Second Fleet in 1790. A number of hypotheses have been advanced concerning the possible source of the epidemic although all are based on the assumption that smallpox was the disease involved.

Tench, writing four years after the epidemic, was one of the first to speculate on the introduction of the disease and in a footnote raised the following questions regarding the origin of the epidemic:

[1] Chickenpox can also be differentiated from smallpox in so far as it is common for eruptions of different stages (age) to exist side by side (that is, vesicles, pustules and scabs), a situation markedly different from that of smallpox.

Is it a disease indigenous to the country? Did the French ships under Monsieur de Peyrouse introduce it? ... Had it travelled across the continent from its western shore, where Dampier and other European voyages had formerly landed? ... Was it introduced by Mr. Cook? ... Did we give it birth here? (Tench, 1979:146)

At the time of writing he had no answers to such questions.

DID IT ACCOMPANY THE FIRST FLEET?

If the disease in question was either smallpox or chickenpox, it is possible that there was an outbreak on the ships of the First Fleet en route to Sydney. Possibly one or more of the vessels involved carried the infection with it and from the settlement it was conveyed to the Aboriginal population, possibly by means of infected clothing or goods or by direct contact. Perhaps again there were some unnoticed or abortive cases of either disease on or after arrival. If the disease in question was chickenpox or very mild smallpox it is possible that the resulting cases went unnoticed or were too mild to excite any comment. Certainly there were circumstances surrounding the medical history of the First Fleet which arouse suspicion. Surgeon White, for example, records in his journal that prior to disembarkation he discovered on the *Alexander* 'a medical gentleman from Portsmouth' who informed him that 'your people have got a malignant disease among them of a most dangerous kind' (White, 1790:2). White inspected those reported to be ill but records no evidence of any malignant disease save a few convicts suffering from inflammatory complaints. Tench, reflecting some time later on the voyage out to New South Wales, implies that there were cases of smallpox during the early part of the voyage when he states: 'no person among us had been afflicted with the disorder [smallpox] since we quitted the Cape of Good Hope' (Tench, 1979:146).

Ross, White and Balmain all refer to a serious outbreak of contagious disease aboard the *Alexander* and how it affected not only the convicts but also the marine detachment. While it is generally accepted that the disease was dysentery (possibly also typhus and/or scurvy) it is possible that cases of smallpox or chickenpox were also present. Certainly it seems more than likely that some of the convicts and the marines must have had personal experience of smallpox before embarkation. Lieutenant Ralph Clark aboard the transport *Friendship*, for example, records in his diary that before sailing for Australia he took leave of his son who was suffering from smallpox (Clark, 1981:12).

Against the view that the ships of the First Fleet brought the disease to Sydney must be set the length of the voyage out, the long period between the fleet's arrival and the appearance of the epidemic, and the comments of Phillip about the absence of smallpox on the voyage. The fleet took 36 weeks to reach Botany Bay including two months from the last port of call, the Cape. This long period would have presumably had a detrimental influence on the survival and infectivity of the smallpox or chickenpox virus. Under optimal conditions, both viruses can remain infective for upwards of a year but are particularly sensitive to ultraviolet light, heat and humidity.

The First Fleet arrived at Botany Bay in mid-January 1788 whereas the epidemic first came to the settlement's attention in early April 1789 — thirteen months later.

If either smallpox or chickenpox was introduced by the First Fleet, it is very hard to understand why no cases came to light in the period after arrival. If it was chickenpox it is possible that the cases of the disease were too mild to excite any interest.

There is also Phillip's report to Lord Sydney of 1790 in which he states that:

> It [smallpox] never appeared on board any of the ships in our passage, nor in the settlement, until some time after numbers of the natives had been seen dead with the disorder in different parts of the harbour. (quoted in Cobley, 1963:141)

Finally, apart from Tench's brief comment there are no other references to smallpox/chickenpox on any of the ships on the voyage to New South Wales.

Clearly some of the ships of the First Fleet suffered considerable sickness on the voyage to New South Wales, particularly the transport *Alexander*. Yet apparently the crew recovered quickly and there is no reason to believe that the illness was caused by smallpox. Despite this it seems certain that there were people aboard the fleet who had had close personal contact with the disease before leaving England.

HMS *SUPPLY* AND NORFOLK ISLAND

A second possible source of infection involves the vessel *Supply*. This ship is implicated because one of its crew, Joseph Jeffries (a native of North America), was the only non-Aboriginal in the settlement to catch the disease. Jeffries manifested the symptoms early in May and died soon after. The *Supply* had returned from a voyage to Norfolk Island late in March. It is possible that Jeffries was exposed to the infection on Norfolk Island and carried it back to Sydney. Against this view is the fact that no record exists of the disease ever visiting the island as well as Collins's comment that Jeffries had previously been to see the two Aboriginal children brought into the settlement suffering from the disease and 'was seized with it soon after' (Collins, 1971:66). Jeffries seems to have visited the children sometime in mid- or late April and the symptoms of the disease appeared on 2 May. (The normal incubation period for smallpox is eight to twelve days with a maximum of fourteen days.)

VARIOLOUS MATTER . . .?

The most tantalizing contemporary comment concerning the possible origins of the epidemic stems from Tench's remark that,

> It is true, that our surgeons had brought out variolous matter in bottles; but to infer that it [the epidemic] was produced from this cause were a supposition so wild as to be unworthy of consideration. (Tench, 1979:146)

What exactly this 'variolous matter in bottles' was, is unfortunately not made clear. There is no mention of such material in 'A List of Medicines for the Use of H.M.

Colony in N.S.W.' dated 12 July 1788 (PRO, CO 201 4:93) nor does there appear to have been any attempt to replenish the supply in ensuing years, if the letters sent back by Surgeon White requesting further medical supplies are any guide.

Yet Tench's reference to 'variolous matter' remains highly suspicious and cannot be dismissed out of hand as the possible source of the epidemic. Inoculation was still the basic method used in 1789 and it was not until the late 1790s that Jenner demonstrated the advantages of vaccination. It is possible that the first surgeons or their assistants attempted to inoculate some of the settlement's population and/or some of the neighbouring Aboriginals and that because of the nature of the matter used and the way it was administered recipients ran the risk of developing anything from a mild to a severe case of smallpox. Further, because attempts to gather and preserve smallpox matter in containers frequently met with mixed success owing to bacterial contamination, side effects and complications would have been common. Razzell, for example, describes the outbreak of smallpox in Boston in the summer of 1800 which resulted from the dispatch of a supply of vaccine from Jenner in London (Razzell, 1977:159). In the Sydney case there is no mention of the variolous matter ever being put to use during the settlement's first year. Yet if the disease was smallpox then this must remain the most likely source of the epidemic. In a recent book, Butlin has canvassed the likelihood of the epidemic originating from this source, postulating an accidental or deliberate infection of the Aboriginal population by the convicts or military authorities. Butlin argues that the outbreak of smallpox could have occurred from (1) accidental infection arising from the bottles containing the variolous matter being stolen or otherwise falling into Aboriginal hands, (2) deliberate attempts by convicts to infect Aboriginals around the settlement, or (3) a calculated campaign of racial extermination carried out by the military authorities (Butlin, 1983:21–2). While Butlin's case largely rests on circumstantial evidence as well as the assumption that the disease agent in question was smallpox it none the less provides a plausible explanation of how the disease might have spread to the Aboriginal population.

WERE THE FRENCH TO BLAME . . .?

Tench's speculation about the epidemic possibly being introduced by La Perouse's expedition was taken up again in 1804 by Thomas Jamison, the colony's principal surgeon, when a notice under his name appeared in the *Sydney Gazette* of 14 October stating that:

> It was generally accredited by the medical gentlemen of the Colony, on its first establishment, that the small-pox had been introduced among the natives by the crews of the French ships then lying in Botany Bay.

From January to March 1788, two ships of La Perouse's expedition had been anchored at Botany Bay where the crews apparently struck up a fairly close rapport with the local natives. There appears to have been no evidence of smallpox among the crew and the epidemic did not break out for at least a year after their departure.

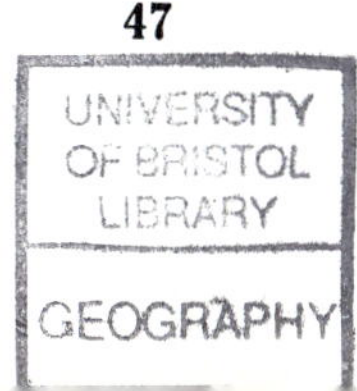

This charge against the French was again revived by Wentworth in the 1820s when he wrote:

> The smallpox, however, at the epoch of the foundation of the colony by Governor Phillip . . . committed the most dreadful ravages among the aboriginal natives. This exterminating scourge was probably introduced by the crews of the vessels of Monsieur de la Perouse, who remained for a short period in Botany Bay . . . and, during his stay there, established an intercourse with the natives; although Captain Cook could not with his utmost endeavours effect this object. As they had, therefore, no communication with the seamen of Cook's vessel . . . it seems that they could only have caught this dreadful pest from the crews of the vessels belonging to this celebrated French Navigator. (Wentworth, 1824:310–11)

It is interesting to compare this statement with an earlier account by Wentworth in 1820 where the same quote is reproduced almost verbatim but with the important substitution of Captain Cook's name for de la Perouse (see Wentworth, 1820:56). As for Wentworth's charge against the French, there seems little supporting evidence. Cleland summarizes the case against such a proposition and dismisses it out of hand (Cleland, 1914:163–70).

WAS IT INDIGENOUS POX?

The claim that the cause of the epidemic was not smallpox but a form of native pox, an infection either introduced many years before or indigenous to the country, originates from Hunter's remark that 'this dreadful disorder, which, there is no doubt, is a distemper natural to the country' (Hunter, 1968:406) and Tidswell's later reflections on the series of local names that the Aboriginals had for the disease, suggesting a long acquaintance with it (Tidswell, 1898).

Speculation surrounding the existence of a form of native pox reached a crescendo during the outbreak of native pox or smallpox in the 1830s and 1840s when many of the colony's medical men debated the nature and origin of the disease prevalent among the Aboriginal population. The evidence is examined by Cumpston who cautiously concludes that:

> the reflections evoked are similar to those . . . relating to other phases of the history of small-pox in Australia, and as it is impossible to overlook the unvarying repetition of the diagnosis of chicken-pox in the cases of the first patients of every epidemic, an uncomfortable feeling is engendered by Dr. Hall's remark that the disease was 'a spurious kind of chickenpox, and was quite as contagious as the other exanthemata'. (Cumpston, 1914:4)

ESTIMATES OF MORTALITY

No detailed information survives on the mortality evoked by the epidemic save a handful of impressionistic contemporary or near contemporary accounts. Most writers seemed stunned by the extent of the mortality even though there seems to have been a tendency to rely on the accounts of friendly natives for estimates of the epidemic's impact on the surrounding Aboriginal population. Collins could write, 'the number that it swept off, by their own accounts, was incredible' (Collins, 1971:597), and to Wentworth the epidemic was an 'exterminating scourge' (Wentworth, 1820:56). The only attempt to estimate the number of deaths comes in a letter written by Phillip to Lord Sydney on 13 February 1790, in which he states:

> It is not possible to determine the number of natives who were carried off by this fatal disorder. It must be great; and judging from the information of the native now living with us . . . one-half of those who inhabit this part of the country died. (*HRA* I, 1:159)

Earlier Phillip had estimated the number of Aboriginals living in the vicinity of the settlement to be in the region of 1500 persons (Phillip to Sydney, 10 July 1788, PRO, CO 201:3). All later comments on the epidemic's mortality draw heavily on Phillip's estimates.

Tidswell, for example, reviewing the epidemic towards the end of the nineteenth century, obviously draws on Phillip's estimate but inflates the geographical extent of the mortality when he writes:

> There is abundant evidence that during its prevalence it produced an enormous mortality amongst the blacks, about one-half of the native inhabitants of *the southern part of Australia* having been killed by it. (Tidswell, 1898:1060, my italics)

Just what this abundant evidence is, is not made clear but it would appear that Tidswell misinterpreted the duration, extent and impact of the epidemic. It would also appear that despite the high mortality the effects of the epidemic may have passed fairly quickly and the local Aboriginal community recovered their numbers. Bradley, for example, records in his journal on 2 June 1789 that 'Twenty Canoes passed Sydney Cove going down the Harbour; this was the first time any number of them had been seen together since the Small Pox having been among them' (quoted in Cobley, 1963:42), and by the end of September there were increasing reports of contact with Aboriginals around the settlement (see, for example, Collins, 1971:81–2). By 1790, the Sydney Aboriginal community seems to have made a remarkable recovery and more than two hundred Aboriginals could gather at Manly to feast on a beached whale (Willey, 1979:111). One is left, therefore, with the feeling that the epidemic was sharp and short-lived and that its effects and extent have been exaggerated out of all proportion.

THE SPATIAL AND TEMPORAL EXTENT OF THE EPIDEMIC

The epidemic appears to have subsided within a month or two. Tidswell, relying on an account given in the *Historical Records* that 'the disease assumed an epidemic character in April 1789 and did not die out until the year 1845', exaggerates the extent and duration of the epidemic when he states 'that an epidemic starting from Sydney in 1789, spread during the succeeding years over the whole of the continent; that it was maintained till 1845, shortly after which it appears to have died out' (Tidswell, 1898:1060). Rather, as Cumpston points out, there were three distinct epidemics of smallpox (or chickenpox) among the Aboriginals. The first, in 1789, affected mainly the Sydney district. The second, in 1829–45, spread from Sydney to a much wider area including the Lachlan, Murrumbidgee, Darling and Murray river systems and possibly further afield, and the third, in 1860–9, which was possibly introduced in the north of the continent, spread in a southwesterly direction (Cumpston, 1914:3). The origin of and relationship between the first two epidemics are largely obscure but each seems to have commenced on the eastern seaboard. The epidemic of 1860–9, which broke out in the Northern Territory and extended into the northern part of Western Australia, appears to have been introduced by Malay fishermen (Cumpston, 1914:3).

The 1789 epidemic originated in or near Sydney in late March or early April and from there made its way up and along the many coves and bays, following the well-used Aboriginal pathways. The disease also diffused in a southerly direction to Botany Bay and up the Georges River. The disease spread a considerable distance along the coast and to its immediate hinterland (Figure 22). Governor Phillip and a party exploring around Broken Bay in June 1789 came across very few Aboriginals and found 'some that had died of the small-pox laying near the path between Port Jackson and Botany Bay'. In September, Hunter, while survey-

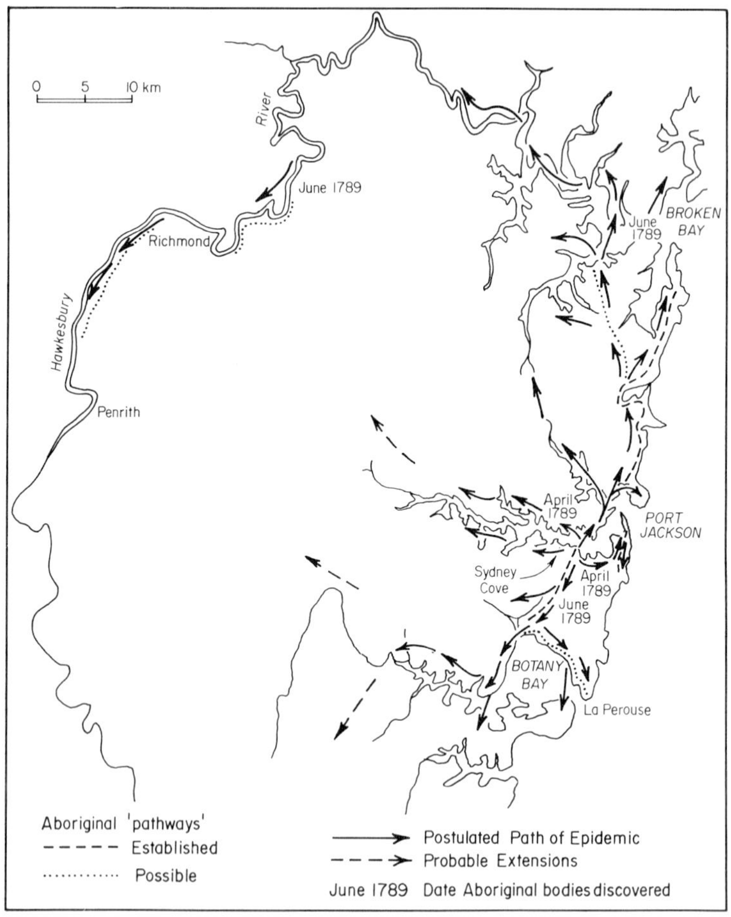

Figure 22 Diffusion of 'smallpox' 1789

ing Botany Bay, discovered human skeletons in some of the caves which he presumed to be smallpox victims. It would seem more than probable that the medium of infection was the Aboriginals themselves as they retreated from the disease. Confronted by a completely unfamiliar disease, they seem to have been terror-stricken and abandoned their sick and fled. Fleeing, they carried the disease with them, as Phillip wrote in 1790:

> and as the natives always retired from where this disorder appeared, and which some must have carried with them, it must have been spread to a considerable distance, as well inland as along the coast. (Phillip to Sydney, 13 February 1790, *HRA* I, 1:159)

Apart from such comments, there is little real evidence to support the view that the disease broke away from its coastal origins and penetrated the interior, even though later writers such as Tidswell and Cumpston were quick to suggest that the epidemic extended beyond New South Wales to Victoria and South Australia. Such assumptions rely on the accounts of early explorers, settlers and doctors who regularly reported contact with Aboriginals bearing the facial scarring of smallpox. All such accounts date from the period 1830–60 and their relevance to the 1789 epidemic would appear highly questionable. Evidence for the epidemic extending beyond the eastern seaboard between Broken Bay and Botany Bay is thus largely circumstantial and difficult to find. There is also a problem regarding the spatial mobility and movement patterns of the Aboriginals inhabiting the Sydney area. In 1789 the coastal Aboriginal people were linguistically, socially and economically distinct from their inland neighbours. There is evidence that the two groups had little knowledge of the life-style and economy of each other, and apart from raiding for marriage partners and some trade there seems little evidence for a mass flight of coastal people into the unfamiliar territory of their inland cousins.[2] More likely, the disease penetrated the interior by virtue of the normal contact patterns between the coastal tribes and their interior neighbours.

TERROR!

The impact of a major epidemic of a disfiguring disease such as smallpox or chickenpox on Aboriginal culture and society must have been profound. Apart from the high mortality, the psychological effect of a disease that struck down only Aboriginals and left Europeans untouched must have been enormous. In addition, a completely unknown disfiguring disease which struck swiftly and within a few days could reduce a healthy individual to an oozing pustulated horror unrecognizable to his close kin or friends must have had a tremendous impact. Those who survived the disease were marked for life physically and psychologically. Wentworth captures some of the fear associated with the epidemic:

> The moment one of them was seized with it was the signal for abandoning him to his fate. Brothers deserted their brothers, children their parents, and parents their children; and, in some of the caves on the coast, heaps of decayed bones still indicate the spots, where the helpless sufferers were left to expire, not so much perhaps from the violence of the disease, as from the want of sustenance. (Wentworth, 1820:56)

[2] See Ross, 1976, for a discussion of the coastal and inland tribes at the time of contact.

WHY WERE NO EUROPEANS AFFECTED?

One of the least explained aspects of the epidemic concerns the contrast between the Aboriginals' apparently extreme susceptibility to the disease and the Europeans' almost universal immunity. It seems amazing that in the face of such a serious epidemic only one immigrant caught the disease. This seems to suggest that the disease may have been present in the settlement but in such a mild or modified form as not to evoke any comment. If the disease was smallpox then it is possible that many had acquired an immunity in Britain where smallpox had been more or less endemic for centuries, particularly in the major towns. By the end of the eighteenth century, smallpox had come to be regarded as just one of a series of common childhood diseases. It is thus likely that most of the officials, marines, sailors and convicts had some prior acquaintance with it or had been inoculated and were at least partially immune. But what of the children born on the voyage or in the settlement? There were approximately fifty such children in the settlement in 1789 and it is surprising despite limited contact with the Aboriginal population that none caught the disease. It is equally surprising that Jeffries was the only non-immune to come into contact with the infection. Even though most adults in the settlement may have had some personal history of smallpox (or chickenpox) we would still expect some variation to exist in their level of immunity; for example, in some people, immunity would not be complete enough to prevent the symptoms of pre-eruptive fever (general fever, head and backache, shivering, sore throat, cough, reddening of the skin plus one or two spots) before the body's immune mechanisms took over to neutralize the virus before it reached the mucous membranes or skin. Unfortunately there is no record of illness in the settlement detailed enough for us to assess whether such symptoms were present, although it is probable that such symptoms may have been simply accepted as commonplace and consequently not thought worth recording. Much the same applies to chickenpox. Mild cases in the settlement may have gone unrecorded as normal day-to-day illnesses.

CONCLUSIONS

Clearly, some sort of epidemic raged exclusively among Sydney's Aboriginal population early in 1789. Whatever the cause and point of origin, it produced at least in the Sydney region a high mortality. Yet was it smallpox? The evidence remains conflicting. A careful reassessment of the documentary sources points as much to chickenpox as to smallpox. The brief description of those suffering from the disease, while generally inconclusive, suggests chickenpox as much as smallpox. The fact that no cases were recorded among the immigrant population suggests that cases of the disease if they did occur must have been extremely mild. Chickenpox seems to have become more or less endemic in Sydney during the 1820s without evoking any public comment and the outbreak of 'pox' in the 1830s and 1840s could easily have been chickenpox.

If the disease involved was smallpox then the questions to be resolved concern the origin of the infection and the means by which it reached the Aboriginal population. It is possible that the origin of the epidemic lay in the government stores of variolous matter and that the virus was somehow loosed upon the Aboriginal population.

It would also appear that the mortality, duration and geographical extent of the epidemic have all been exaggerated. From Phillip's assessment of 50 per cent mortality in the Sydney region, Tidswell projected the mortality level to involve the whole of southeastern Australia. The epidemic also seems to have disappeared within a few months and the outbreak of the disease which became apparent after 1829 was a new epidemic. Finally, the evidence for the epidemic extending well beyond Sydney into the interior and beyond is, to say the least, highly suspect.

We shall probably never know what disease caused the high mortality among Sydney's Aboriginal population in 1789 nor exactly how it was introduced. Yet an epidemic did take place and caused substantial mortality and disruption, although whether it caused, in the words of Willey, 'a crippling loss of numbers from which events . . . gave them no chance to recover' (1979:78) is highly doubtful.

CHAPTER FOUR

'Count Your Children'

The Measles Epidemic of 1867

Count your children after the measles has passed.
Arabic proverb

INTRODUCTION

DISEASES such as smallpox and bubonic plague have left their indelible mark upon the course of human history. The effect of measles, by contrast, was much more subtle, particularly in the role it played in the mortality of young children during the nineteenth century. During the nineteenth and early twentieth century people tended to be more afraid of diseases such as scarlet fever and diphtheria, and the merest hint of plague or smallpox was enough to excite considerable panic. Measles, by comparison, was accepted as commonplace. To many people in Sydney, measles was regarded much as it is today, generally a mild disease of infancy, a short-term nuisance. One rarely fears what is everyday and familiar and for the most part so little deadly. For many, however, particularly those of Sydney's poor, the situation was somewhat different, and where conditions of poverty and/or depressed living conditions prevailed and where children were malnourished (especially where there was a protein deficiency) measles was often a much more prolonged and severe disease leading to high case fatality rates. The same applied where the disease was introduced into virgin soil or where the infection had become unknown for a generation or more. In such circumstances the results could be catastrophic. Measles was, therefore, viewed differently by Sydney's residents and the effect that the disease had upon the city during the latter half of the nineteenth century vividly illustrates the wide gulf that existed between Sydney's upper and lower classes. The full impact of the disease during the nineteenth century is, however, obscured if one relies simply on the number of deaths occurring under its name. Throughout this period the loss of weight and emaciation associated with an attack of measles was a considerable influence on the mortality of young children and many deaths occurring from diarrhoea, dysentery and broncho-pneumonia were triggered by an attack of measles. The interaction of measles, malnutrition and other infections remained particularly close throughout this period. Also, unlike today when measles reaches a peak in children soon after they begin to socialize in preschool and primary school (that is, 3–5 years of age), in the nineteenth century the infection occurred mainly in the home environment and at a younger age (1–3 years).

The 1867 measles epidemic, while not the first outbreak of measles of major proportions in Sydney, related to all these truths. This epidemic stands as a clearly defined event in Sydney's social and epidemiological history and ushered in a period when measles was to play an important role in morbidity and mortality. The 1867 outbreak represented the most severe childhood epidemic of the nineteenth century and it is possible to infer from the severe mortality accompanying the outbreak that many families in Sydney were living in marginal conditions with children suffering some degree of protein deficiency and malnutrition. While the infection rate was probably high in all social classes it was the poor who suffered the heaviest mortality. It would also appear that children raised in poor families in crowded and depressed surroundings contracted the disease at a younger age and were more likely to suffer complications leading to death.

That such a severe epidemic should have evoked almost no public comment or concern seems surprising to the twentieth-century observer. Yet given the general perception of the disease and the fact that Sydney's more vocal and articulate upper and middle classes were spared the worst effects of the epidemic, it is perfectly explicable.

MEASLES: THE DISEASE

Measles then as now remains one of the most ubiquitous and persistent of human viruses. It is typically an acute highly contagious childhood disease characterized by fever, conjunctivitis, cough and general skin eruptions. A single attack produces life-long immunity. Since the virus commonly inhabits the upper respiratory tract, dissemination is by droplet spread and the disease spreads quickly in the home, school or institutional environment. Within such situations the disease spreads progressively and as each child passes through an infectious phase and becomes immune the virus finds it increasingly more difficult to spread and must await the arrival of a new crop of susceptible children before the cycle can repeat itself. A striking feature of measles in nineteenth-century Sydney was its periodicity, its recurrence in epidemic form at regular intervals. Measles outbreaks tend to occur in distinct waves, often with a regular interval separating epidemic peaks. In Sydney from mid-century measles epidemics established a periodicity of between five and eight years (Table 11). There would seem to have been several factors involved in determining this interval. In order for an epidemic to occur, the proportion of the population who were immune needed to fall below a critical level. The proportion of susceptible children was determined by new generations coming into contact with the virus for the first time and was then governed by a variety of socio-economic conditions, particularly living conditions, child nutritional levels

Table 11 Periodicity of Measles Epidemics, Sydney 1834–98

Epidemic year in Britain		*Epidemic year*	*Previous free interval (years)*
1838–50[a]		1834–5	?
		1854	19
		1860	6
1866	⟶	1867	7
1874	⟶	1875	8
		1880	5
1887	⟶	1888	8
		1893	5
1898	⟶	1898	5

Sources: Parish Registers; Creighton, 1965; Cumpston, 1927; Donovan, 1970; Jamieson, 1908.
[a] Measles more-or-less endemic.
⟶ Indicates possible interconnection.

and the socialization process of infants determined in part by such things as family size, schooling and institutional life. A certain population size was also necessary to sustain the disease in an endemic pattern within any community. Normally this has been taken to be in the region of 250 000 persons. Sydney did not reach a population of this magnitude until the 1880s and consequently it would seem that measles was continually reintroduced from overseas rather than maintained as an endemic infection. Epidemics normally faded out when the numbers of susceptible children were exhausted or too few to allow the maintenance of successful chains of transmission. In such a manner did measles epidemics occur in nineteenth-century Sydney and come to play a vital role in the city's social and epidemiological life.

HISTORY OF MEASLES IN SYDNEY

In Europe throughout the eighteenth century and the early years of the nineteenth century, there were frequent measles outbreaks with a widespread prevalence after 1830. It is not surprising, therefore, that Australia should have had some experience of the disease early in its period of settlement. The first ship to arrive at Sydney bearing a history of measles on the voyage arrived in 1829. The first epidemic, however, occurred five years later with the arrival of the *David Scott* on 25 October 1834 (Donovan, 1970). This epidemic extended into the following year and spread well beyond Sydney as far as the South Island of New Zealand where it caused terrible mortality among the Maori population (Hocken, 1898:51). By the 1850s measles would appear to have become well-established in Sydney, whether endemic or continually reintroduced by the many shipping arrivals remains a matter of dispute. By this date Sydney's population had increased to approximately 80 000 and that of New South Wales to 270 000. A more severe epidemic of measles broke out in the city in March 1854 and although no official records exist the burial registers of Camperdown Cemetery clearly show a considerable surge of mortality in the months of March and April when 285 deaths

Table 12 Deaths, Camperdown Cemetery, January–June 1853–6

	Jan.	*Feb.*	*March*	*April*	*May*	*June*
1853	83	93	58	67	93	68
1854	94	92	162	123	79	73
1855	106	73	90	88	74	71
1856	104	70	52	69	69	41

Source: Camperdown Cemetery Burial Registers, 1853–6.

occurred, two and a half times the average for the two-monthly period in preceding and ensuing years (Table 12). Almost 67 per cent of these deaths were under five years of age. As further evidence, the records of the Sydney Dispensary indicate that 57 people sought treatment for measles in 1854.

During the 1850s many of the ships arriving at Sydney had a record of measles and other infectious diseases on the outward voyage. The *Beejapore*, for example, possibly responsible for the 1854 epidemic, sailed from Liverpool with 1023 passengers in 1853 and on arrival at Sydney was quarantined for 54 days after measles and scarlet fever had broken out on the voyage. All in all, 124 passengers died, including 106 children, between the time the vessel left Liverpool and when it finally berthed at Sydney (Cumpston, 1927:236). Such a pattern repeated itself throughout the 1850s. At least twenty ships were quarantined on arrival at Sydney between 1853 and 1860 after a history of measles on the trip out. Sydney's third measles epidemic occurred in 1860 and was responsible for 272 or 10 per cent of the city's total deaths in that year. Eighty-three per cent of all those who died from the disease during this year were under five years of age. Seven years later Sydney suffered its worst epidemic when the disease again broke out and in only a handful of months carried off more than 700 young children.

For the 50 years after 1854 measles continued to be one of the most important infectious diseases of children in Sydney. Whether it became endemic before the 1880s remains a matter of conjecture but the close relationship between epidemic years in Australia and Britain seems supportive evidence in favour of a periodic reintroduction hypothesis. Whatever the point of origin there is little doubt as to the amount of suffering and mortality caused by the disease in the latter half of the nineteenth century.

THE 1867 EPIDEMIC

On 6 February 1867 Annie Jennings, the three-year-old daughter of a Balmain storekeeper, died of measles. Her death was to usher in the most catastrophic childhood epidemic Sydney has known. Most people alive in 1867 could remember the measles and influenza epidemic of 1860 when in a short space of time more than 360 people, mostly young children, had died. Few were prepared for a repeat performance seven years later when in a little over five months measles swept away more than 700 young children. Although we have no way of knowing just how many people caught measles and survived in 1867 it would appear that the infection rate was very high. Possibly as many as 13 000 young children caught the disease in this year and if this figure is anywhere near accurate then

70 per cent of all Sydney's young children under five years of age must have had measles. Whatever the actual number of cases there can be no disguising the severity of the outbreak. Clearly it was a disaster to rank alongside the influenza epidemic of 1919 in Sydney's history.

THE TEMPORAL-SPATIAL DIFFUSION OF THE EPIDEMIC

Annie Jenning's death took place early in February but it was not until some weeks later that it finally became evident that Sydney was poised on the brink of a period of unusual morbidity and mortality. From mid-February the number of deaths rose rapidly from 14–20 per week to more than 60 by late March/early April. The peak of the epidemic was reached in a six-week period between late March and the first week of May (weeks 7–12, Figure 23). During this short period measles raged in Sydney with great virulence and more than 370 young children were carried off by the disease. More than 50 per cent of all deaths during the epidemic occurred in this six-week period. The epidemic continued unabated into the beginning of May but by the second week there were signs that it was losing its momentum. From more than 40 deaths a week in early May, the number fell to below 20 by June and to less than 10 by the following month. Between 20 February and 4 June 667 deaths or 89 per cent of all epidemic deaths had occurred.

Within Sydney, particular residential areas showed some variation in their temporal pattern (Figure 24). In Brisbane and Gipps wards, for example, the epidemic both peaked and declined earlier, achieving its maximum mortality during March and falling rapidly away thereafter. In nearby Phillip, by contrast, peak mortality occurred later, in mid-April to early May. Within the metropolitan area, Balmain and The Rocks area exhibited the earliest onset of deaths followed by Brisbane and Denison wards and the two central wards of the City (Bourke and Macquarie). Generally, the epidemic appeared earliest in the western and central parts of the

Figure 23 Temporal distribution of measles epidemic 1867

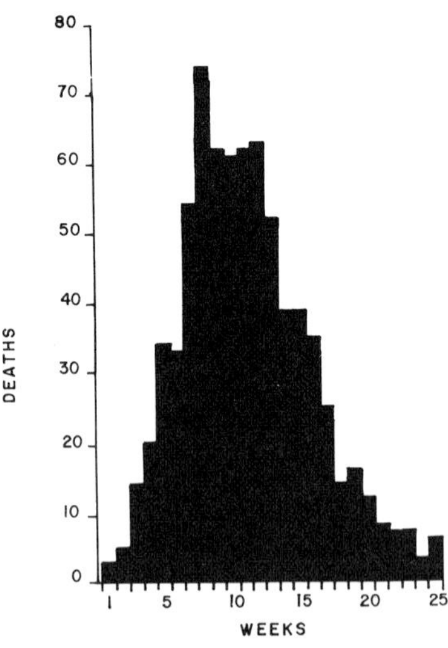

City and from there spread in all directions, in some cases bypassing suburbs like Paddington only to gather them up at a later date (Figure 25). By the middle of March the epidemic had engulfed, in addition to the City of Sydney, North Sydney and St Leonards on the North Shore, the inner western suburbs of Glebe, Camperdown and Redfern, Woollahra and Randwick to the east and St Peters to the south. From here it penetrated southwards to Botany, caught up suburbs previously bypassed such as Paddington and Lane Cove, and extended as far as Five Dock, Rockdale and Parramatta (Figure 25).

The peak period of mortality (based on highest weekly death totals) is not as regular as the pattern of onset. Generally, the period of highest mortality occurred earliest in Gipps and Brisbane wards and in the municipalities of St Leonards, St Peters and Camperdown. The areas affected latest (Rockdale, Marrickville, Five Dock, Petersham and Parramatta) all experienced late peaks of mortality. Some areas, however, such as Denison, Phillip and Fitzroy, experienced relatively late periods of peak mortality despite the early onset of the disease. The following broad pattern thus emerges. For outer suburban areas measles arrived late and departed fairly early. For other areas the onset was early, the peak late and the duration of the epidemic prolonged. Figures 26 and 27 by mapping the fortnightly

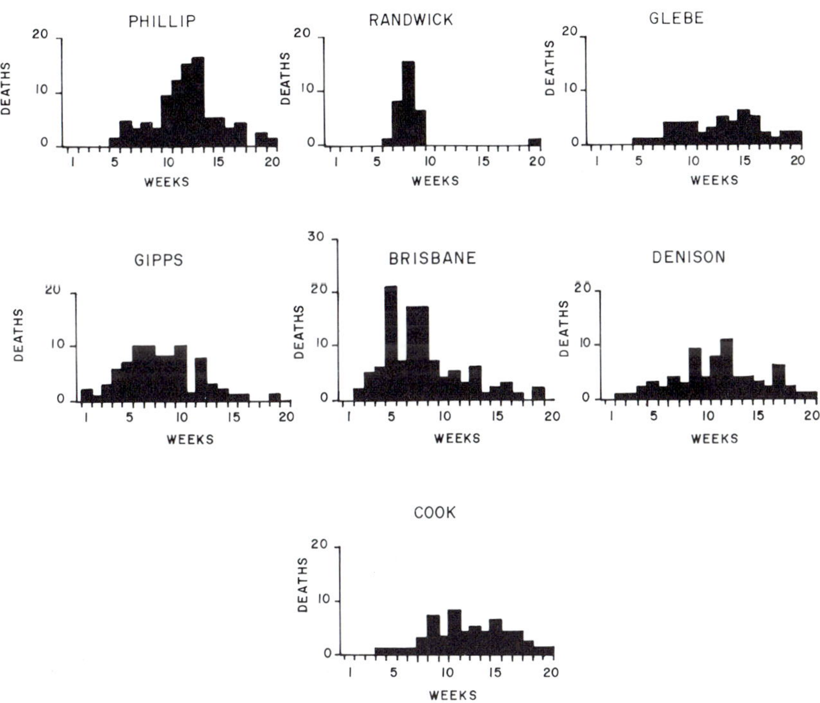

Figure 24 Temporal distribution of measles epidemic, selected Sydney wards and suburbs 1867

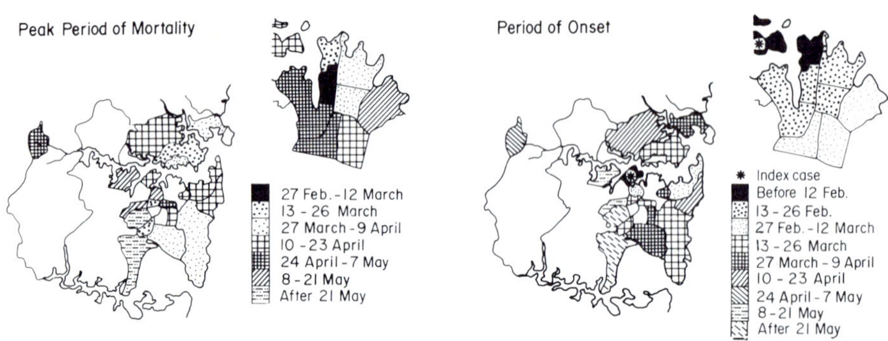

Figure 25 Onset and peak mortality of measles epidemic 1867

progression of deaths provide a general summary of the disease's spatial diffusion through Sydney. These maps support the points made above and show measles spreading from its original focus to engulf the city and surrounding suburbs.

SPATIAL DISTRIBUTION

Unfortunately no evidence exists as to the number or areal distribution of cases of measles during the epidemic. If we can infer the spatial incidence of the disease from the deaths that occurred under its name then the epidemic was spatially highly concentrated, occurring chiefly in the City of Sydney and the two inner western municipalities of Balmain and Glebe. Seventy per cent of all measles deaths occurred within the boundaries of the City of Sydney alone, the majority of which were concentrated within a belt of closely packed working-class residential neighbourhoods extending from the lower Rocks to the Haymarket (Figure 28). The three wards bordering Darling Harbour contributed 36 per cent of all deaths, and as Figure 29 illustrates, the bulk of these were in three spatial clusters: (1) the lower Rocks area between Cumberland and George Streets; (2) Sussex and adjacent streets between Bathurst and Erskine Streets; (3) the north end of Pyrmont about John, Harris and Church Streets.

For the remainder of the City, most deaths took place in the western fringe of Woolloomooloo, the northwestern part of Surry Hills and at the Benevolent Asylum in Phillip ward. Outside the City, only Glebe, Balmain, Randwick and Woollahra recorded more than 20 deaths. Interestingly enough some of the innermost suburbs of Sydney seem to have escaped the worst aspects of the epidemic. Leichhardt and Newtown, for example, experienced no deaths while Camperdown, Petersham and Marrickville had only a handful.

The area that suffered the heaviest mortality comprised all the City of Sydney with the exception of the central ward of Bourke, the eastern ward of Fitzroy, and the municipality of Glebe (Figure 28). More than 500 deaths occurred within this area, approximately 68 per cent of all deaths in the epidemic.

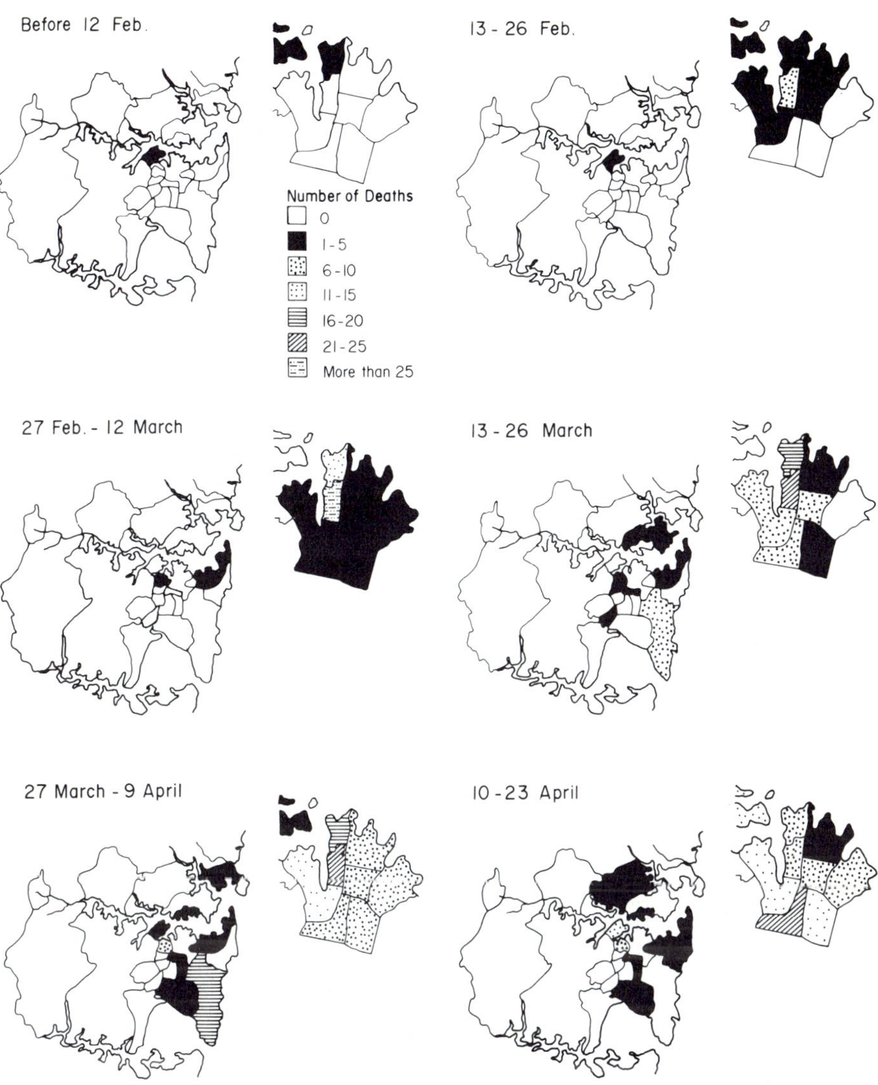

Figure 26 Spatial diffusion of measles epidemic, February–April 1867

CHAINS OF TRANSMISSION

The epidemic was complex because transmission took place in a variety of locales: within the household, in the streets and yards between neighbours or visitors, within institutions, and probably within churches and schools. There were 48 cases of multiple deaths in the household (111 deaths in total), indicating that within-household spread of the disease accounted for 15 per cent of the total

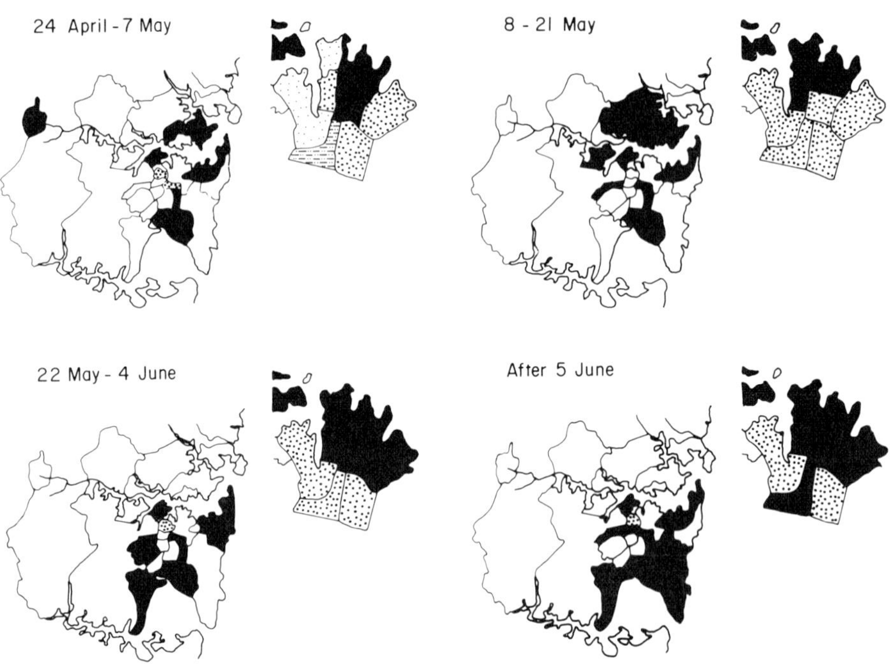

Figure 27 Spatial diffusion of measles epidemic, April–June 1867

deaths. Institutions accounted for 80 of the 748 deaths (11 per cent).[1] Neighbourhoods, that is contact in the street or lane, in the home of friends and neighbours or across the backyard, were the location of three-quarters of all transmissions. Most chains of contagion occurred between persons from houses sharing a cesspit or sanitary convenience, a washing basin or tap, or from personal contacts centred on the street or backyard. It was in these locales that personal contacts between members of different households most frequently took place. The process of contagion is perhaps best described as a series of mini-epidemics which swept through the crowded working-class residential areas in central Sydney progressing from household to household along particular streets.

MORTALITY

The 1867 epidemic provides us with some idea of the mortality that could accompany a measles epidemic in the mid-nineteenth century. Between mid-February and the end of July there were 748 deaths from measles within the Sydney urban area, representing more than one-fifth of all Sydney's deaths for the year. In the City of Sydney the impact of the epidemic was even greater, account-

[1] Seventy-seven deaths occurred in the Benevolent Asylum and Destitute Children's Asylum, two cases in the Victoria Barracks and one at the Darlinghurst Gaol.

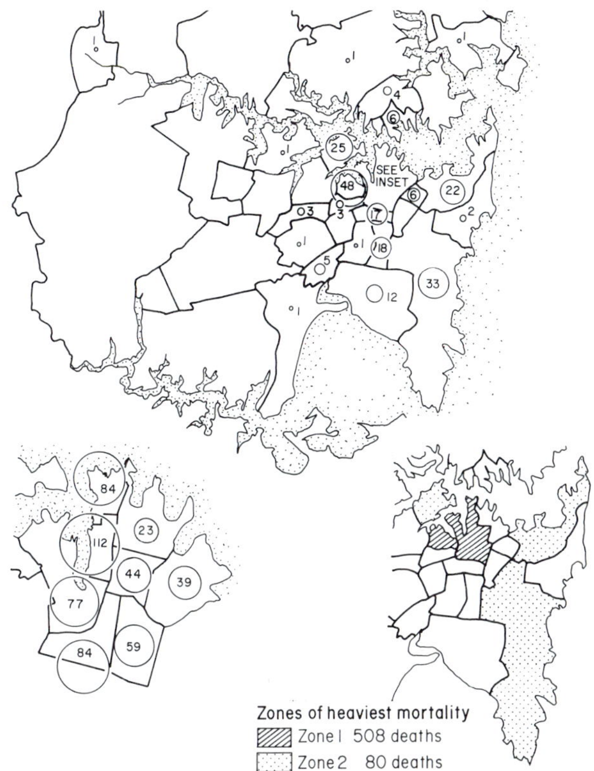

Figure 28 Distribution of measles deaths, metropolis 1867

ing for almost one-quarter of the annual number of deaths. When child deaths alone are considered, however, the full impact of the outbreak becomes clearer. Almost half of all deaths between the ages of one and five years in 1867 were caused by the measles epidemic (Table 13). Within the City of Sydney the epidemic caused substantial disruption to the lives of the inhabitants. In Brisbane ward, for example, 55 per cent of the year's death came during the epidemic and in three other wards the proportion was between 29 and 37 per cent (Table 14).

Clearly this was a disaster of major proportions. When the crude death rate from measles is mapped (Figure 30) it shows the differential spatial impact of the epidemic upon the city. The outbreak was at its severest in Brisbane ward, Randwick and Botany, followed by Phillip ward. When the death rate is made more age-specific and considers measles deaths per 1000 aged one to seven years, much the same pattern emerges with the death rate being highest in Brisbane ward (96.8), Randwick (92.7) and Botany (80.0).

AGE AND SEX INCIDENCE

As Figure 31 graphically illustrates, the epidemic mainly affected Sydney's infant population, particularly those aged between one and four years. Overall almost 80

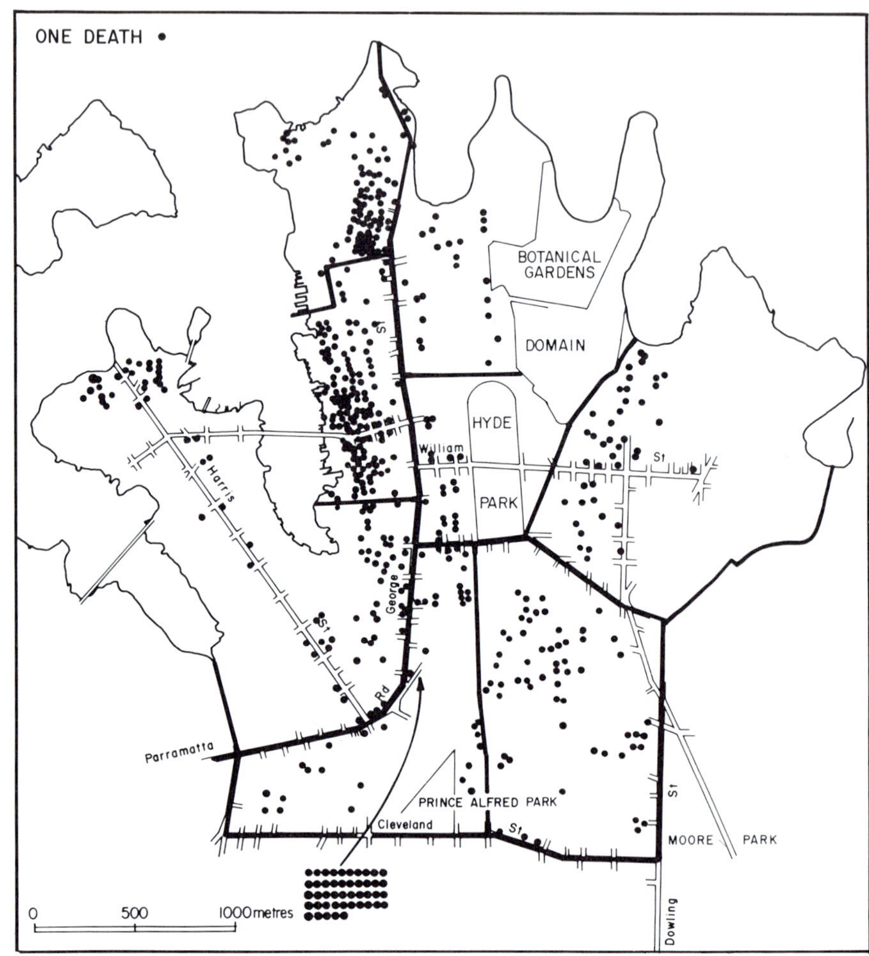

Figure 29 Distribution of measles deaths, City of Sydney 1867

Table 13 Measles Deaths, Sydney City and Metropolitan Area 1867

	Total deaths	*Measles deaths*	*Deaths 1–5 yrs*	*Measles deaths 1–5 yrs*	*Deaths 1–10 yrs*	*Measles deaths 1–10 yrs*
Sydney City	2151	552 (24.3)[a]	797	394 (49.0)[b]	904	487 (46.4)[c]
Sydney Metropolitan Area	3537	748 (21.2)[a]	1318	646 (49.4)[b]	1524	707 (53.9)[c]

Sources: Registrar-General, Death Records; Vital Statistics, 1867.
Note: These figures apply only to measles deaths occurring during the epidemic period and not the whole year, thus understating the full impact of measles deaths on total deaths in 1867.
[a] Measles deaths as a percentage of total deaths.
[b] Measles deaths aged 1–5 as a percentage of total deaths 1–5 years.
[c] Measles deaths aged 1–10 as a percentage of total deaths 1–10 years.

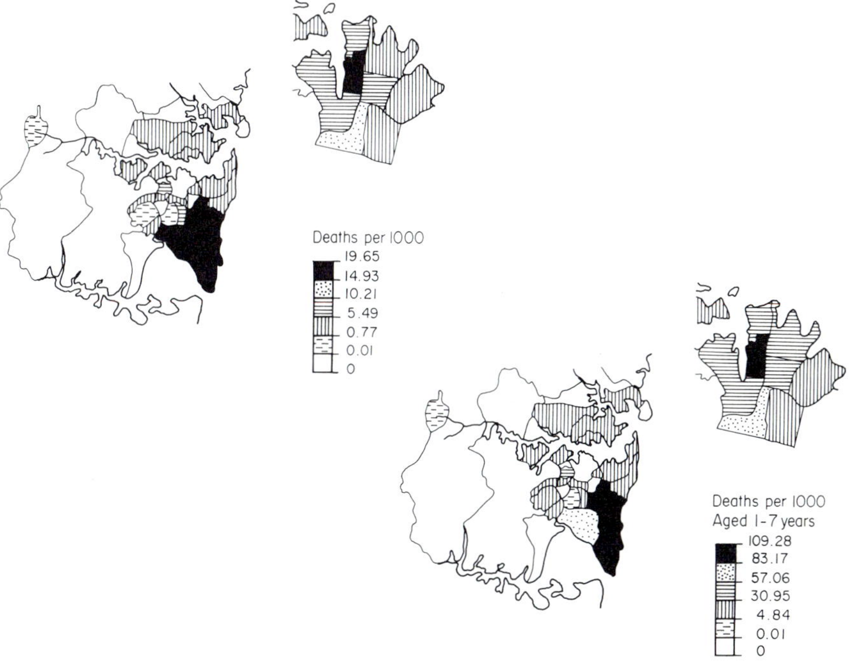

Figure 30 Crude and age-specific death rates, measles epidemic 1867

per cent of all deaths were aged between one and four years with a further 14 per cent aged from five to eight years (Figure 31). Very few deaths occurred in infants under one year, because of the immunity-transfer of antibodies *in utero* from the mother, or to children over nine years. The age structure of deaths faithfully reveals the type of epidemic it was, that is, a family-neighbourhood centred outbreak affecting mainly young children at home. Only in the case of

Table 14 Measles Deaths as a Proportion of Total Deaths, City of Sydney Wards 1867

City ward	*Measles deaths*	*Total deaths*	*Measles deaths as % of total deaths*
Gipps	84	285	29.5
Brisbane	112	202	55.4
Denison	77	263	29.3
Phillip	84	257	32.7
Bourke	23	396	5.8
Macquarie	44	116	37.9
Cook	59	242	24.4
Fitzroy	39	390	10.0

Sources: Registrar-General, Death Records; Vital Statistics, 1867.

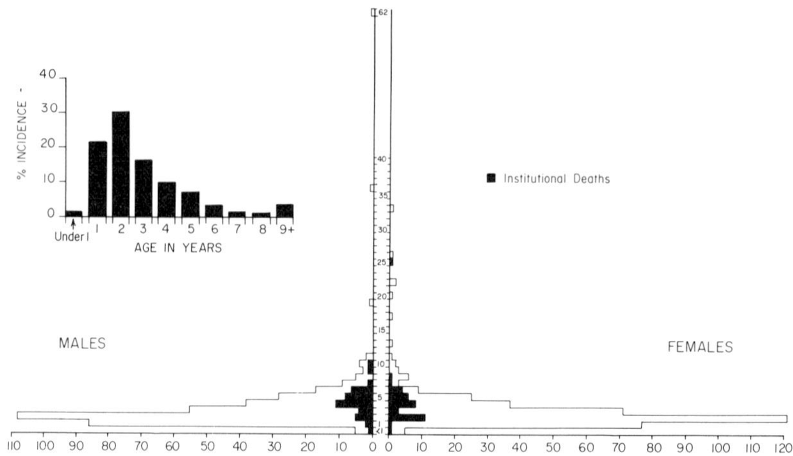

Figure 31 Age-sex incidence of measles deaths 1867

Sydney's institutional population were children over five years of age at risk.[2] As Table 15 and Figure 31 illustrate, a much greater proportion of institutional deaths were in the 5–8 age group (35 per cent compared with 11 per cent of non-institutional deaths). In the case of the 1–4 age group, the proportion of institutional deaths was 58 per cent compared to a figure of 82 per cent for the remainder of the population.

Chapin's classic 1925 study of more than 141 000 measles victims in Providence, Rhode Island demonstrated the attack rate to be highest in the sixth year, or first year of school life. One-quarter of all cases studied by him occurred by the end of the second year of life, half by the end of the fourth year and three-quarters by the end of the sixth (Chapin, 1925). By comparison the mortality of the Sydney epidemic of 1867 showed a much more youthful age structure, particularly among the non-institutional population. Fifty-seven per cent of deaths had occurred by the end of the second year, 83 per cent by the end of the fourth and 91 per cent by the end of the sixth. Such an age distribution suggests a number of things: (1) that the infection occurred chiefly in the home and immediate neighbourhood environment, that is, among a group of susceptibles characterized by a low degree of spatial mobility; (2) that the spatial organization of central city tenements characterized by crowded living conditions, close-knit household groups, extensive neighbouring and shared recreational and sanitary facilities led to greater occasions for contact and helped channel the spread of the disease; and (3) that the social and spatial framework of the institutional population contributed to the spread of the disease.

SOCIO-ECONOMIC STATUS

In terms of mortality the epidemic was particularly severe on Sydney's disadvantaged classes. Whereas the infection rate was probably high among all social

[2] The two institutions concerned were the Benevolent Asylum and the Randwick Destitute Children's Asylum.

Table 15 Age-Sex Structure of Deaths, Measles Epidemic 1867

	Non-institutional			*Institutional*[a]			*Total*		
ge group	*Males*	*Females*	*Total*	*Males*	*Females*	*Total*	*Males*	*Females*	*Total*
-1	4	4	8	1	1	2	5	5	10
-4	265	283	548	22	23	45	287	306	593
-8	44	31	75	15	12	27	59	43	102
-15	7	7	14	2	—	2	9	7	16
6+	3	6	9	—	1	1	3	7	10
ot stated	5	12	17	—	—	—	5	12	17
otal	328	343	671	40	37	77	368	380	748

urce: Registrar-General, Death Records, 1867.
Benevolent Asylum, Randwick Destitute Children's Asylum.

groups the likelihood of serious illness and/or death depended very largely on the health and nutritional status of the child. Consequently Sydney's poorest families were the hardest hit. Table 16 lists deaths by the socio-economic status of the household head. Immediately apparent is the contribution that Sydney's lower classes made to the epidemic. Taken as a group, the unskilled/semi-skilled, asylum, destitute and illegitimate population accounted for almost half of all deaths. Many of the remainder, however, were the children of tradesmen differentiated from the former group not so much by their affluence or better living conditions as by their possession of some small skill or trade, the majority working for themselves as bootmakers, carpenters, butchers, smiths and printers. Together these two broad groups made up 81 per cent of all measles deaths in 1867.

Few of Sydney's middle and upper classes were seriously affected by the epidemic. Only a handful of clerical and professional parents lost children. On the other hand, 82 deaths occurred to the children of small businessmen/proprietors — 11 per cent of all deaths. The majority of such people were grocers, store-

Table 16 Deaths from Measles by Socio-economic Status, 1867 Epidemic

Socio-economic class[a]	*Number*	*%*
Unskilled	226	30.2
Semi-skilled	64	8.6
Small tradesmen	236	31.5
Clerical, etc.	9	1.2
Small businessmen/proprietors	82	11.0
Professional/gentlemen	6	0.8
Army	3	0.4
Asylums[b]	77	10.3
Pauper	1	0.1
Illegitimate	5	0.7
Not stated	39	5.2
Total	748	100.0

Source: Registrar-General, Death Records, 1867.
[a] In most cases this refers to the socio-economic status of the father.
[b] Benevolent Asylum, Randwick Destitute Children's Asylum.

keepers, innkeepers and dealers who by the very nature of their business either lived cheek-by-jowl with Sydney's lower classes or regularly came into contact with them in the course of business or recreation.

COMPLICATIONS

In just under 50 per cent of cases the actual cause of death was from complications following or associated with an attack of measles. In severe cases of measles all the epithelial surfaces of the body including the respiratory and gastrointestinal tracts are affected and may lead to severe complications (Morley, 1980:122). In the young child this may manifest itself as bronchial pneumonia or in the case of the gastrointestinal tract as enteritis or diarrhoea. Such was the case in the 1867 epidemic. The most common complications (Table 17) were gastrointestinal (diarrhoea, dysentery, other gastrointestinal) followed by broncho-pneumonia. These two groups accounted for 52 per cent of all complications. The only other categories to figure prominently were other childhood infections such as diphtheria, croup, whooping cough and scarlet fever. The state of nutrition appears to affect the epidemic behaviour of the disease. Protein deficiency particularly seems to be associated with a much higher incidence of complications, especially broncho-pneumonia and diarrhoea, and a severe attack of measles itself can accentuate the effects of malnutrition on the child (Morley, 1980) (Figure 32). It would appear likely, therefore, given the young age groups affected by the epidemic and the high proportion of complications leading to death, that a high level of malnutrition existed among many of Sydney's infants in 1867.

THE MINI-EPIDEMICS

The Benevolent Asylum run by the Benevolent Society, a private charity supported by the New South Wales government, opened its doors in 1821 on a site at the

Table 17 Complications Associated with Measles Deaths, 1867 Epidemic

	Number	*%*
Broncho-pneumonia[a]	88	24.2
Diarrhoea/dysentery	77	21.2
Other gastrointestinal	23	6.3
Convulsions	38	10.4
Childhood infections[b]	56	15.4
Effusion/congestion of brain	30	8.2
Typhoid	9	2.5
Other fever	8	2.2
Dentition	8	2.2
Other	27	7.4
Total	364	100.0

Source: Registrar-General, Death Records, 1867.
[a] Inflammation and congestion of lungs, bronchitis, pneumonia.
[b] Diphtheria, croup, whooping cough, scarlet fever, meningitis.

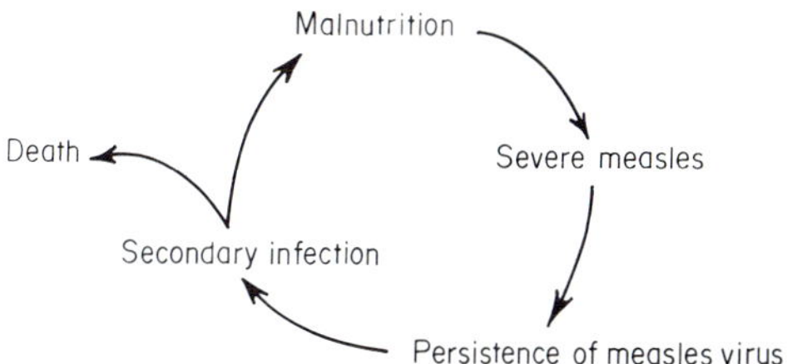

Figure 32 Malnutrition-measles cycle

southern end of the town where the Central Railway Station now stands.[3] Initially its purpose was to provide relief and shelter to Sydney's most disadvantaged and pauperized groups as well as institutional and medical care for the chronically ill and infirm. The Society also provided outdoor relief to needy families. Basically the Asylum was divided into two broad sections, a chronic diseases infirmary and a workhouse where able-bodied inmates were expected to work. In the 1850s the Asylum underwent a change in function, partly as a response to increasing pressure on its resources. In 1851 the Society took over the temporary use of the Liverpool Hospital and transferred most of its male inmates to Liverpool. Thereafter the Asylum was restricted to females and their children and to orphan children over the age of eight years. In 1862 the government took over the care of the aged, destitute and infirm, and four years later the north wing of the Asylum was set aside as the Lying-in Hospital of New South Wales, catering mainly for poor mothers-to-be. The proportion of children admitted to the Asylum varied during the 1860s according to the demands on the Society's orphan school and the asylum at Paddington. At the time of the epidemic the Asylum offered accommodation to approximately 70 women and 200 children.

The Society for the Relief of Destitute Children was formed in 1852 with the express aim of providing accommodation for Sydney's abandoned and destitute children under the age of eight years. The Society occupied a building on a 60-acre site at Randwick in 1858 with accommodation for approximately 400 children. Later this accommodation was expanded to provide room for an additional 400 children. At the time of the measles epidemic the Society had approximately 500 children in care at Randwick, the majority between the ages of four and ten years.

Throughout the 1860s the Benevolent Society acted as a filter for destitute children. The sick, ailing and physically imperfect remained at the Asylum while the others were sent to the Randwick institution. In 1867 both these institutions, in so far as they provided an organizational framework which brought together large numbers of young children in an enclosed environment, offered a fertile breeding ground for the spread of infectious disease.

The year 1867 was crucial for both institutions. During March, Sydney experienced an outbreak of whooping cough which in a few weeks caused high morbidity and mortality among young children. The Randwick Destitute Children's Asylum lost 32 children from the disease and the Benevolent Asylum more than

[3] For a discussion of the origin and early development of the Benevolent Society, see Cummins, 1971.

20. Worse was to follow for in the next two and a half months measles swept through both institutions attacking many of the inmates and causing high mortality. The epidemic broke out first in the Destitute Children's Asylum and if deaths resulting are indicative of the temporal frame of the outbreak then the epidemic was sharp and short-lived. Commencing on 19 March (week 6), it was virtually over within four weeks (Figure 33). The peak was reached in the week commencing 27 March and most children died in the two-week period between 20 March and 2 April. In all, 31 young children died from measles during the epidemic. Most were aged between four and seven years and all but one died from secondary complications (mostly diarrhoea and exhaustion) suggesting some degree of nutritional deprivation.

The annual medical report for the year confirms the health status of the children who died. In the words of the report 'the children attacked were invariably the

Table 18 Age-Specific Mortality Rates, Destitute Children's Asylum 1867 (measles deaths per 100)

Age (years)	*Males*	*Females*	*Total*
3	25.0	0.0	5.5
4	23.5	13.3	12.5
5	17.5	10.0	13.7
6	13.9	2.5	7.9
7	3.1	4.2	3.6
8	0.0	3.1	1.6
9	5.0	0.0	2.2
10	4.5	0.0	2.4
3–10	9.9	5.9	7.0

Sources: Registrar-General, Death Records, 1867; Randwick Asylum for Destitute Children, Register of Inmates.

Table 19 Age-Sex Structure, Institutional Deaths, Measles 1867

Age	*Destitute Children's Asylum*			*Benevolent Asylum*			*Total*		
(years)	*Males*	*Females*	*Total*	*Males*	*Females*	*Total*	*Males*	*Females*	*Total*
0–1	—	—	—	1	1	2	1	1	2
1	—	—	—	2	1	3	2	1	3
2	—	—	—	5	11	16	5	11	16
3	1	—	1	3	3	6	4	3	7
4	4	4	8	7	4	11	11	8	19
5	7	4	11	1	2	3	8	6	14
6	5	1	6	1	3	4	6	4	10
7	1	1	2	—	—	—	1	1	2
8	—	1	1	—	—	—	—	1	1
9	1	—	1	—	—	—	1	—	1
10	1	—	1	—	—	—	1	—	1
25	—	—	—	—	1	1	—	1	1
Total	20	11	31	20	26	46	40	37	77

Source: Registrar-General, Death Records, 1867.

weakest and most impoverished in constitution' (Coulter, 1916:23). The report further stated that those most susceptible to the infection were 'infants of three years, often scrophulous or syphilitic . . . yet free from contagious disease' (ibid.). Tables 18 and 19 provide some indication of the mortality during the epidemic. Generally four-, five- and six-year-olds suffered most heavily, although in the case of males three-year-olds shared the heavy mortality.

The children resident in the Benevolent Asylum suffered even more severely from the epidemic although in this case the outbreak did not strike until some weeks later. The first recorded death from measles took place on 11 April (week 10) and the last on 22 June (week 16) but for all sense and purposes the epidemic was concentrated in an eight-week period between 11 April and 4 June (Figure 33). During this period 45 young children succumbed to the disease, the majority in a two-week period between 24 April and 7 May. By comparison with the Destitute Children's Asylum a smaller proportion of the deaths at the Benevolent Asylum were due to secondary complications and most of these were from other childhood infections such as croup, whooping cough and typhoid.

These two institutional mini-epidemics invite comparison. In so far as both institutions led to a spatial clustering of susceptible population, they played an important part in the rapid spread of the disease. The outbreak at the Destitute Children's Asylum occurred earliest, largely affected 4–6-year-olds (reflecting the population at risk) and evinced a high degree of secondary complications indicating marginal health conditions among the inmates. The outbreak at the Benevolent Asylum by contrast occurred two weeks after the finish of the Destitute Children's Asylum's epidemic and extended much later. Here mortality was much heavier, the children affected younger (mainly 2–4-year-olds), and there were fewer secondary complications.

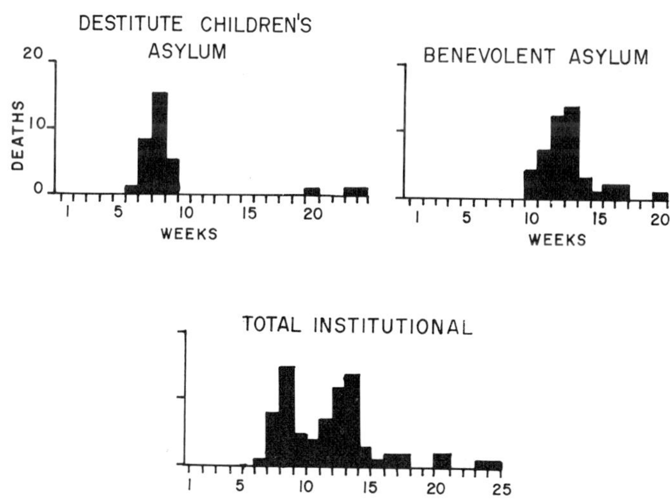

Figure 33 Temporal distribution of measles deaths in Sydney institutions 1867

CONCLUSIONS

The measles epidemic of 1867 was probably the greatest childhood disaster of the nineteenth century. Possibly as many of 70 per cent of all young children in Sydney caught the disease during May and June 1867 and more than 700 were swept away by it. By all accounts this was a great morbidity and mortality crisis which had a tremendous impact on families living in the central part of Sydney. While the infection rate was probably high in all social groups it was the city's poor who suffered the greatest mortality. To this extent the epidemic was indicative of the high degree of malnutrition that existed among families in inner Sydney. It is interesting to speculate what impact this malnutrition had on reproductive capability and whether or not there was any resulting decrease in fertility. The greatest irony surrounding this epidemic was that despite its severity it evoked little or no public reaction and was largely accepted as a commonplace incident of childhood.

CHAPTER FIVE

The Dreaded Scarlet Fever

The Epidemic of 1875–6

THE TERM scarlet fever or scarlatina has been known in English for centuries. During the nineteenth century Sydney's inhabitants held the disease in particular dread for it conveyed much more of a sense of contagion and drama than did measles, which was largely accepted as a normal incident of childhood. Perhaps this was because the disease was particularly virulent in Sydney or perhaps because 'scarlet' is an emotive word. Certainly the disease was responsible for a great amount of human suffering in the last half of the nineteenth century. Scarlet fever was also one of a number of diseases which varied in their virulence over the last few centuries. In Britain the disease was particularly deadly during the eighteenth century and then assumed a milder form between 1800 and 1830 before it increased in severity again. Between 1845 and 1876 the disease reached such virulence as to cause Creighton to remark: 'The enormous number of deaths from Scarlatina during the thirty or forty years in the middle of the nineteenth century will appear in the history as one of the most remarkable things in our epidemiology' (Creighton, 1965:726). After 1876 the disease entered another mild phase long before the advent of sulphonamide (1930s) or penicillin treatment (1940s). It would appear that neither curative or preventive medicine nor improved living conditions, hygiene or diet played any role in this decline and that change in the incidence and virulence of the disease owes more to biological factors, particularly the interaction between host and virus.

HISTORY OF SCARLET FEVER IN SYDNEY

Scarlet fever was probably first introduced to Sydney by immigrant ships in the late 1830s. Records indicate that both the *John Barry* and the *Maitland*, which arrived in Sydney in 1837 and 1838 respectively, were quarantined on arrival after outbreaks of the disease on the voyage (Cumpston, 1927:180). The first reference to cases of the disease among Sydney's population occurred two years later in 1840 when the annual report of the Sydney Dispensary records ten people seeking treatment. A further five patients were also treated at the Benevolent Asylum in the same year. The first epidemic probably commenced late in 1840 and continued into the following year. The annual report of the Sydney Dispensary records 69 cases of scarlet fever treated in 1841. By the 1850s the disease had become well established in the city, whether endemic or periodically reintroduced remains arguable although the coincidence of epidemics in England with those in Sydney seems to offer strong support for the reintroduction hypothesis. After 1850 and particularly in the 1860s and 1870s scarlet fever became one of the most significant childhood diseases in Sydney and the cause of much suffering. Like measles, outbreaks of the disease adopted a particular periodicity related in the main to outbreaks in Britain. As Table 20 indicates, the interval between outbreaks generally varied from four to eight years between 1840 and 1900.

After 1876, as in Britain, the disease entered a milder phase and while epidemics still occurred (as in 1893 and 1898) there were fewer deaths than previously. Cleland estimates there to have been approximately 2000 cases of the disease in Sydney in the first half of 1893 with 149 deaths, representing a case fatality rate of 7.45 (Cleland, 1911:244), whereas by the 1898 epidemic 2425 cases produced only 32 deaths, a case fatality rate of only 1.03 (Cumpston, 1927:464). Between 1898 and 1901 the case fatality rate for the disease in Sydney varied between 1.03 and 1.80. Unfortunately little evidence exists for the earlier period. The incidence of the disease seems to have varied throughout the nineteenth century from 0.5 to 5.2 cases per 1000 in normal years to about 50.0 per 1000 in epidemic years. The records of the Sydney Dispensary for the years 1841–65 provide some evidence of the incidence of the disease but nothing on its virulence. In 1841–2 for example, there were 2.1 cases of the disease per 1000 of Sydney's population, in 1850 1.3 and in 1864 only 0.5. In 1898 there were 5.1 cases per 1000 in Sydney, 1.2 in 1899 and 0.9 in 1900.

THE 1875–6 EPIDEMIC

The epidemic of scarlet fever which broke out in Sydney during late September 1875 and extended into the first half of 1876 was part of a much wider epidemic which affected New South Wales, Victoria, South Australia and Tasmania and caused more than 5000 deaths. The epidemic differed in many respects from the catastrophic outbreak of measles of eight years previous. In the first place, it extended over a much longer time period. In the second, its effects were spread over a wider geographical area. In the third place, it produced a wave of public reaction and a widespread concern for public health and sanitation. The epidemic lasted for approximately 40 weeks during which time it caused more than 570 deaths. In the period following the measles epidemic there had been important changes in Sydney's geography and social structure. The intervening years had seen a rapid increase in suburban population and a related decline in the numbers living within the City of Sydney. There had also been increasing socio-economic differentiation of Sydney's workforce. The scarlet fever epidemic related to both these developments. Spatially the epidemic was much more concentrated in

Table 20 Periodicity of Scarlet Fever Epidemics, Sydney 1840–98

Epidemic year in England		*Epidemic year*	*Previous free interval (years)*
1840	⟶	1840–1	?
1848	⟶	1849–50	8
1858–9	⟶	1858–9	8
1863–4	⟶	1863–4	4
1874	⟶	1875–6	7
		1893	17
		1898	5

Sources: Parish Registers; Sydney Dispensary, *Annual Reports*; Creighton, 1965; Cumpston, 1927; Jamieson, 1908.
⟶ Indicates possible interconnections.

Sydney's inner suburbs than in the central city and whereas the measles epidemic had mainly affected the children of Sydney's unskilled/semi-skilled population the scarlet fever outbreak tended to affect a greater proportion of the city's middle- and upper-class families. Finally, the epidemic engendered considerable public concern and led to a series of official reports investigating the origin, prevalence and means of transmission of the disease.

SCARLET FEVER IN 1875–6

In 1875–6 the cause and means of transmission of scarlet fever were unknown. It was widely believed that the germs of specific poisons which caused the disease were always present in the densely settled parts of a city and that they just required the right set of environmental circumstances to burst forth in epidemic proportions. The disease began then as now with a rapid rise in temperature, soreness and redness of the throat, and eventually a generalized macular rash of intense red colour on the chest and limbs. After a few days the temperature fell and the skin began to peel. In most cases the patient was ill for several days with a sore throat, high temperature, fever and loss of appetite. Medical practitioners in Sydney during the epidemic were of the opinion that the disease was spread by 'minute poisonous atoms which came off the body of the sick through the skin, bowels and kidneys and from the membranes of the lungs, throat and nostrils' (Health Society of N.S.W., 1876:3). In an effort to stop the spread of the disease doctors were urged to anoint the sufferer's body with either suet, lard or olive oil so as to affix the poison-charged particles to the body (see Wilson, 1927:353–5). The beneficial nature of this treatment was recommended on the grounds that the fats not only mechanically fixed poisons to the body but also combined with oxygen to form peroxide of hydrogen, 'a substance remarkable for its power of destroying zymotic poisons' (ibid.:354). Otherwise doctors recommended a regime of magnesium sulphate, quinine sulphate, ferrous sulphate, diluted sulphuric acid and belladonna. The epsom salts was to clear out the bowels, the quinine served as a nerve tonic, the iron as a blood stimulant, the diluted sulphuric acid as an antiseptic and the belladonna was to quieten the reflex action of the nerves. For the throat a gargle of potash and hydrochloric acid was also recommended, supplemented in severe cases by a poultice of camomile flowers and regular massaging of the chest and throat with soap liniment, turpentine and belladonna.

TEMPORAL DISTRIBUTION

Although the epidemic probably began in late September or early October 1875 it was not until a month later that people in Sydney became aware that a major outbreak of scarlet fever was under way. From the second week of November until June of the following year Sydney suffered the ravages of a particularly virulent outburst of scarlet fever. The epidemic came in two major waves, the last followed by a lull and then a brief reprise.

After a slow start the first wave ushered in a period of high mortality extending from early November (week 7, Figure 34) to the end of January (week 18). This twelve-week period produced 236 deaths, 41 per cent of all deaths during the epidemic. The second wave, more prolonged than the first, began at the beginning of February (week 19) and extended until the third week of May (week 34). During this sixteen-week period 248 deaths occurred, 43 per cent of all deaths in the epidemic. This was followed by a fall in the number of deaths until late June when there was a short reprise. By mid-July the epidemic was over.

Some parts of Sydney suffered equally during the two waves. This was true of the City of Sydney, particularly Cook and Fitzroy wards, as well as Paddington and Redfern. The first wave tended to be concentrated in the western suburbs of the city, particularly in a belt of suburbs extending in a southwesterly direction from Redfern to Canterbury. The second wave mainly affected Balmain, Glebe, Redfern, Waterloo, Paddington, Woollahra and several suburbs on Sydney's North Shore.

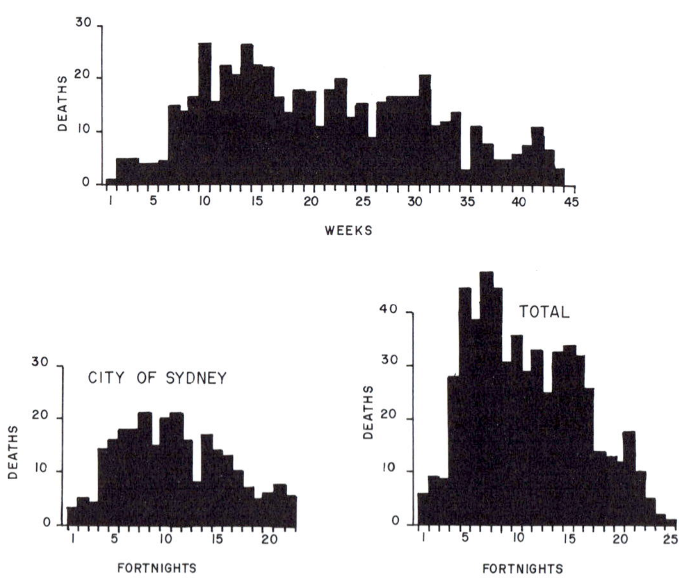

Figure 34 Temporal distribution of scarlet fever deaths 1875–6

Figure 35 illustrates the temporal progression of the epidemic in a series of City wards and suburbs. Newtown provides a good example of a suburb affected mainly by the first wave. Here the epidemic was sharp and relatively short-lived, being virtually over by the end of January. Balmain and Glebe, by contrast, were primarily affected by the second wave of the epidemic and deaths were concentrated in the period after February.

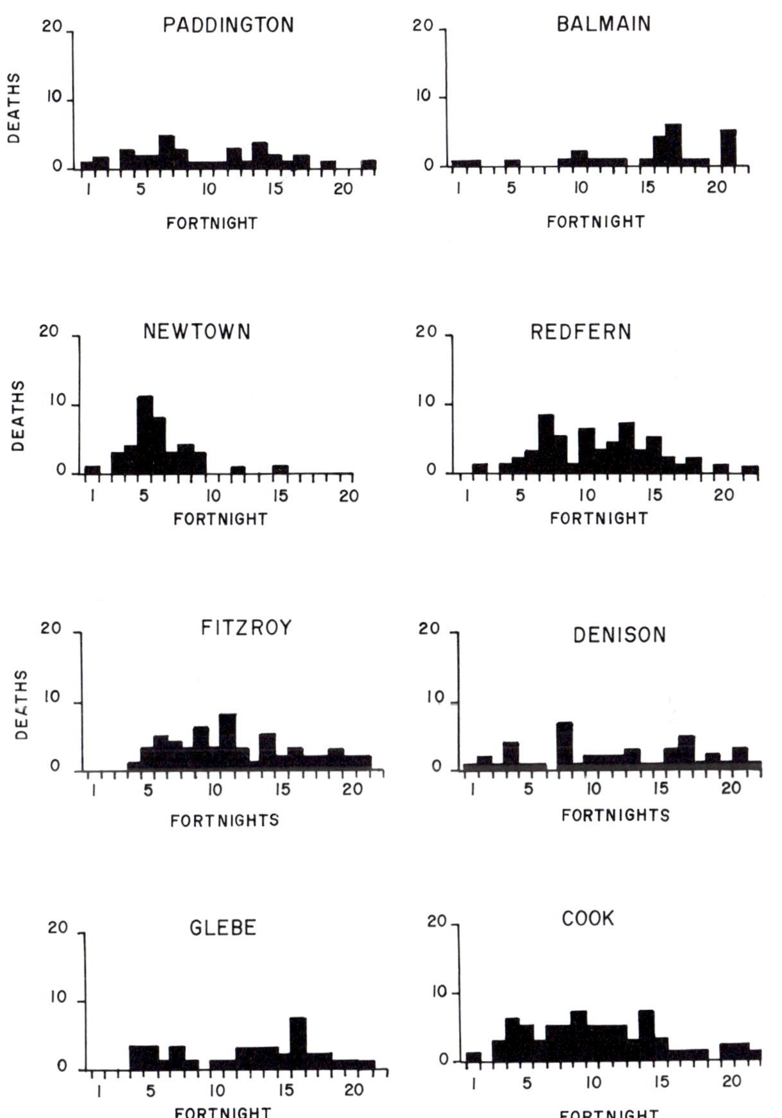

Figure 35 Temporal distribution of scarlet fever deaths, selected wards and suburbs 1875–6

Figure 36 shows the date of onset for the various parts of the Sydney urban area. The epidemic first appeared in Newtown and within a week deaths had also occurred in Balmain, Paddington and in parts of the City of Sydney. By the end of October the epidemic was virtually confined to the City of Sydney (excluding Bourke and Fitzroy wards) and to the four inner municipalities of Balmain, Paddington, Redfern and Newtown. During the next few weeks the epidemic slowly spread to encompass Fitzroy in the City, Petersham and Glebe in the west, Woollahra in the east and crossed the harbour to Victoria (North Sydney). The next month saw a major southeastward extension of the disease to engulf the municipalities of Marrickville, Alexandria, St Peters, Canterbury, Rockdale and Hurstville. Finally, the epidemic increased its foothold on Sydney's North Shore by penetrating Hunters Hill, Lane Cove, St Leonards, Mosman and Manly.

Interestingly, some areas could remain unaffected for long periods as the epidemic raged about them. Fitzroy and Bourke wards in the City, for example, remained untouched until November despite the experience of the rest of the City. Waterloo remained unaffected until late March, Waverley until mid-January. A general overview of the epidemic's diffusion across Sydney can be obtained by mapping the fortnightly progression of deaths (Figures 37–39). These maps support

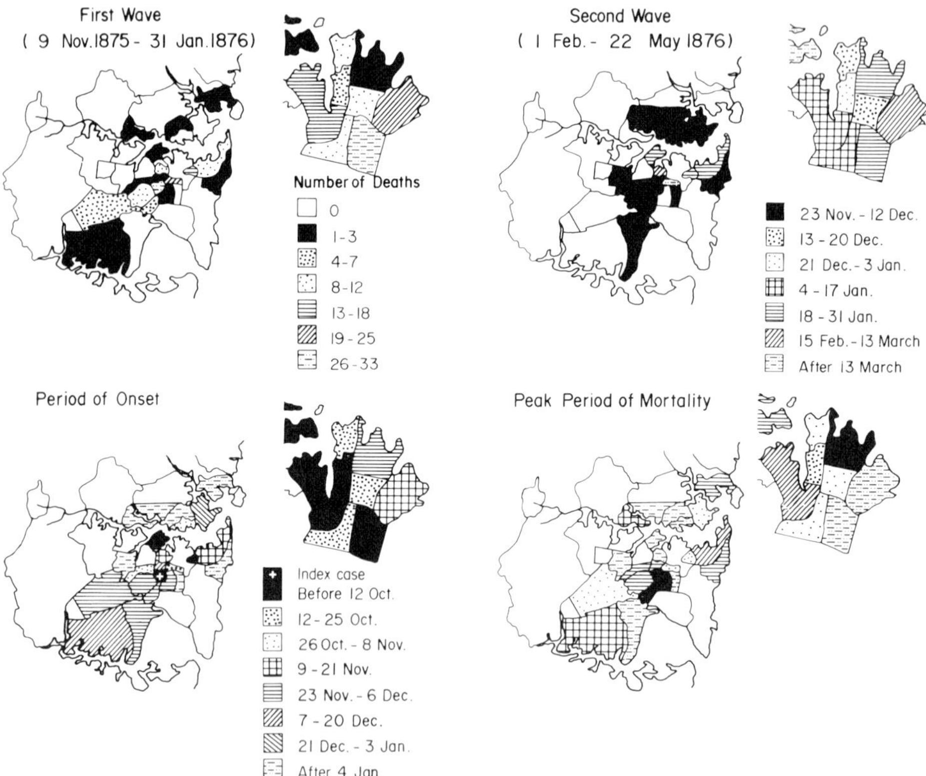

Figure 36 Diffusion waves, onset and peak mortality, scarlet fever epidemic 1875–6

the points made above. The broad pattern up until the end of the first wave (31 January) shows the epidemic peppering the City of Sydney and inner suburbs and gradually spreading to involve the western and southwestern suburbs. During the second wave the disease remained concentrated in the City of Sydney, the northern and eastern suburbs but also penetrated to the southern suburbs of St Peters and Rockdale.

Figure 36 reveals the period of highest mortality to have occurred earliest in the three inner suburbs of Newtown, Alexandria and St Peters and latest in the outer

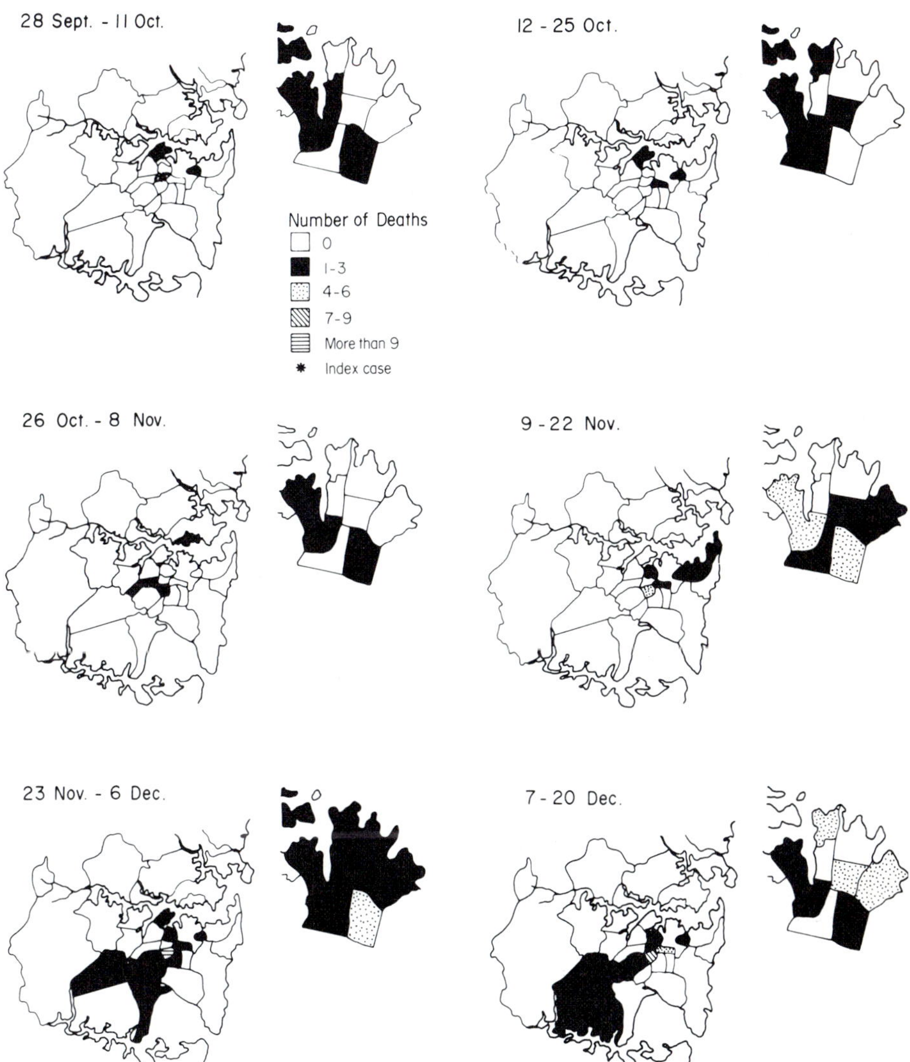

Figure 37 Diffusion patterns, scarlet fever epidemic, September–December 1875

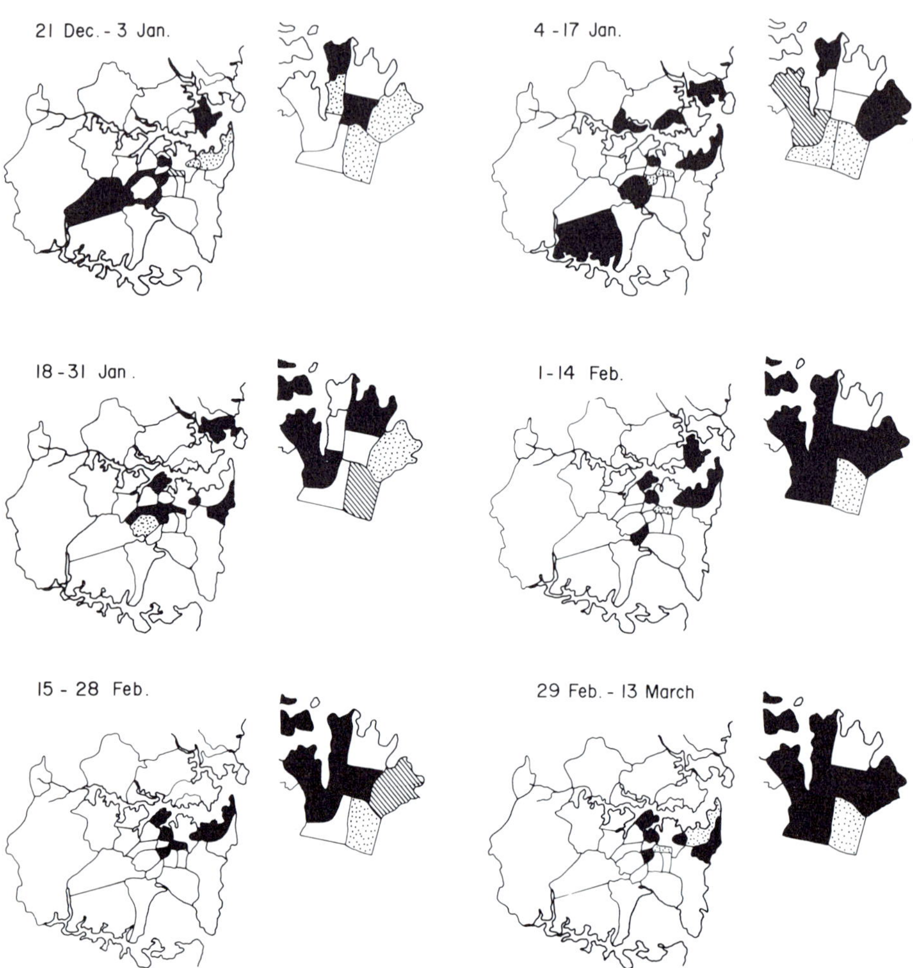

Figure 38 Diffusion patterns, scarlet fever epidemic, December 1875–March 1876

suburban areas of St Leonards, Lane Cove, Ashfield and Rockdale. There were some notable exceptions to this pattern, however, and those inner suburbs that mainly participated in the second wave, such as Balmain, Glebe and Waterloo, all experienced a late peak in mortality. The City of Sydney reveals a different pattern. Gipps, Brisbane and Macquarie wards showed the earliest peak, followed by Denison and Phillip, with Bourke, Cook and Fitzroy experiencing the latest.

SPATIAL DISTRIBUTION

The geographical distribution of deaths from scarlet fever during the 1875–6 epidemic largely reflected the spatial distribution of Sydney's population and in par-

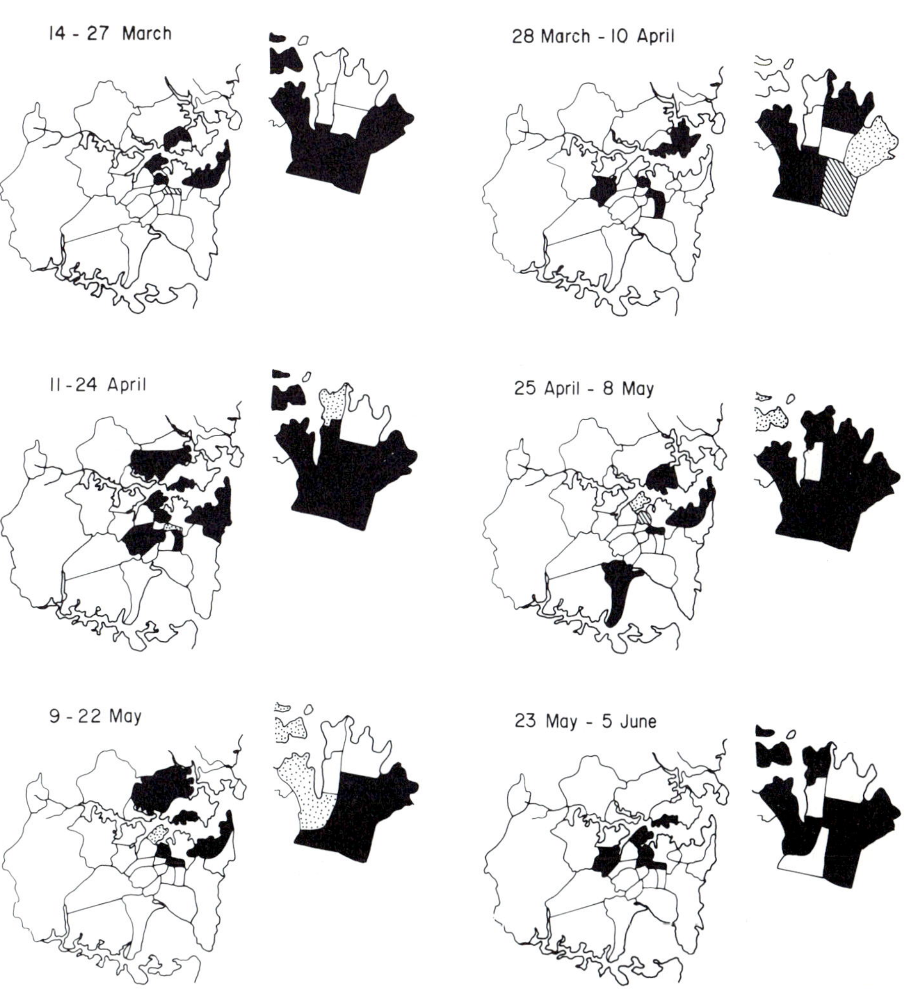

Figure 39 **Diffusion patterns, scarlet fever epidemic, March–June 1876**

ticular the changes in that pattern that had taken place in the previous ten years. By 1875–6 approximately 48 per cent of Sydney's population lived within the boundaries of the City of Sydney compared with approximately 56 per cent eight years earlier. The biggest change had taken place in the innermost suburbs surrounding the City which by 1875–6 housed approximately 37 per cent of the total urban population. In 1867 the proportion living in the inner suburbs had been closer to 25 per cent. Deaths during the epidemic mirrored these distributional changes. Forty-six per cent of all deaths occurred to people resident within the City of Sydney and 38 per cent to those in the inner suburbs. The remainder were confined to the more peripheral residential areas. As Figure 40 reveals, spatially the epidemic was concentrated in three major areas of the city. The first area of

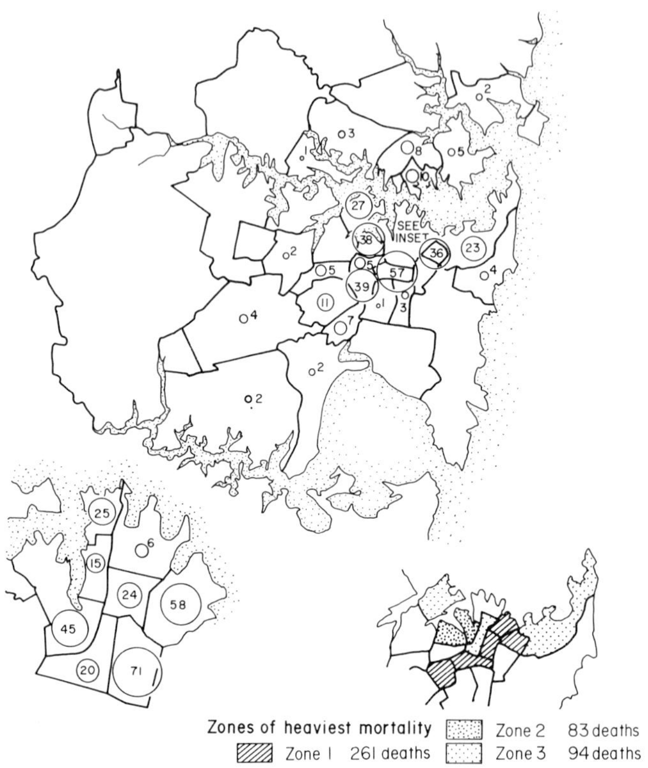

Figure 40 **Distribution of scarlet fever deaths 1875–6**

concentration was an inner-city residential belt extending from Paddington in the east through Kings Cross, Woolloomooloo, Darlinghurst and Surry Hills to Redfern and from there to Newtown. More than 45 per cent of all deaths occurred within this broad zone. A second spatial concentration of scarlet fever deaths was to be found in a group of disadvantaged residential areas extending from the Haymarket, Ultimo and Pyrmont to Glebe. This area contributed approximately 14 per cent of all deaths. Finally, there were four discontinuous areas of high mortality comprising the central wards of Phillip and Macquarie and the municipalities of Balmain and Woollahra which contributed a further 16 per cent of deaths. Together these three broad areas accounted for more than three-quarters of the epidemic's total mortality. Some areas escaped the worst effects of the epidemic almost entirely. No scarlet fever deaths were recorded in Leichhardt, Botany or Randwick and only a handful in Alexandria, Waterloo, Rockdale and the northern suburbs. In terms of the spatial distribution of deaths the epidemic invites comparison with the measles outbreak of 1867. In the case of the earlier outbreak 80 per cent of all deaths took place in the City of Sydney, Balmain and Glebe; in 1875–6 only 57 per cent of scarlet fever deaths were recorded in these areas.

MORTALITY

Between September 1875 and late July 1876 the epidemic claimed the lives of 575 people, the majority infants under the age of five years. This mortality represented approximately 15 per cent of all deaths that took place in Sydney over the epidemic period. The impact on Sydney's infant population was even more marked. Three-quarters of all epidemic deaths were aged under five and these deaths represented almost one-quarter of all infant deaths that took place in Sydney during the period September to July. In particular areas of the city the epidemic's demographic impact was even greater. In the City of Sydney, for example, more than 16 per cent of all deaths between October and July were from scarlet fever and in the period December–April the proportion was consistently in excess of 20 per cent (Table 21).

Figure 41, which shows the death rate per 1000 persons aged one to seven years, provides some indication of the spatial impact of the epidemic on the lives of Sydney's infant population. Mortality was highest in a belt of residential suburbs stretching from Woollahra and Paddington in the east through the eastern residential areas of the City of Sydney (Fitzroy and Cook wards) to Redfern, Newtown and Marrickville and from there to Ashfield, Canterbury, St Peters and Rockdale. In the north another belt of high mortality took in the North Shore suburbs of Victoria (North Sydney), St Leonards and Mosman. In the inner west, Glebe also shared in this high mortality. Within this overall area, the mortality rate among infants was highest in Paddington, Newtown, Marrickville and Victoria.

Regrettably no record has been left of the number of cases of scarlet fever during the epidemic. Assuming a case fatality rate of between 5 and 7.5 per 100 then there must have been approximately 8000 to 10 000 cases of the disease in Sydney.

Table 21 Scarlet Fever Deaths, City of Sydney, October 1875–July 1876

Month	*Scarlet fever deaths*	*Total deaths*	*Scarlet fever deaths as % of total deaths*
1875			
October	6	139	4.3
November	26	158	16.4
December	43	199	21.6
1876			
January	40	194	20.6
February	37	159	23.3
March	33	162	20.3
April	40	170	23.5
May	16	167	9.6
June	11	139	7.9
July	12	148	8.1
Total (Oct.–July)	264	1635	16.1

Source: Registrar-General, Death Records, 1875–6.

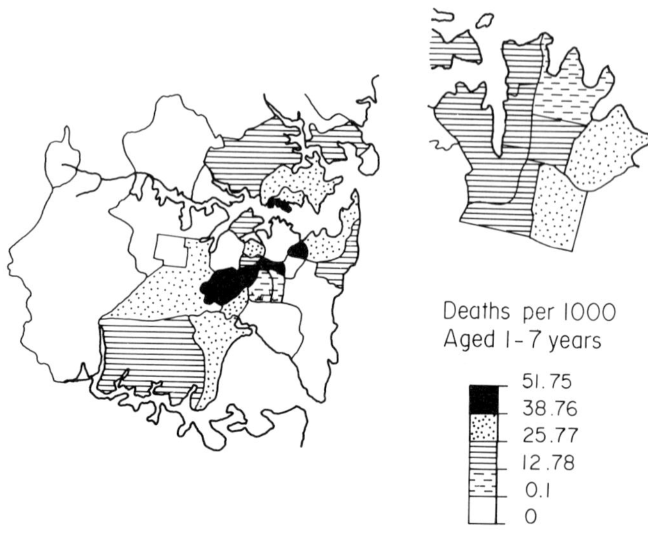

Figure 41 Death rate per 1000 aged 1–7 years, scarlet fever epidemic 1875–6

AGE-SEX DISTRIBUTION

Figure 42 and Table 22 illustrate the age-sex distribution of deaths during the epidemic. Like the earlier measles outbreak the scarlet fever epidemic was almost exclusively concentrated among Sydney's infant and young child population with almost 80 per cent of total deaths being aged 1–7 years. Two-thirds were aged under 5 with the majority 1–4 years. The effects of this particular epidemic in terms of the age groups affected were more wide-ranging than the measles outbreak. Almost 15 per cent of deaths were, for example, aged over 8 years including 11 per cent between the age of 8 and 18 years. In summary, the age distribution of deaths was approximately 6 per cent under one year, 60 per cent aged 1–5 years, 28 per cent from 5 to 14 and 3 per cent aged 15–24 years. The higher proportion of older children and teenagers suggests that the epidemic spread within families and that older children were often as much at risk as younger ones. After 1876 it appears that the age distribution of cases and deaths from scarlet fever shifted away from the young infant groups to include a greater proportion of 5–14-year-olds (see Gandevia, 1978:87).

SOCIO-ECONOMIC STATUS

Table 23 details the social class of the breadwinner of families who lost a child or children during the epidemic. Once again the unskilled/semi-skilled sector of Sydney's population suffered heavily although in this case only one-third of all deaths came from this group. The children of Sydney's middle and upper classes seem to have been more heavily affected by the scarlet fever outbreak than they had been by the measles epidemic of eight years before. Over one-quarter of all

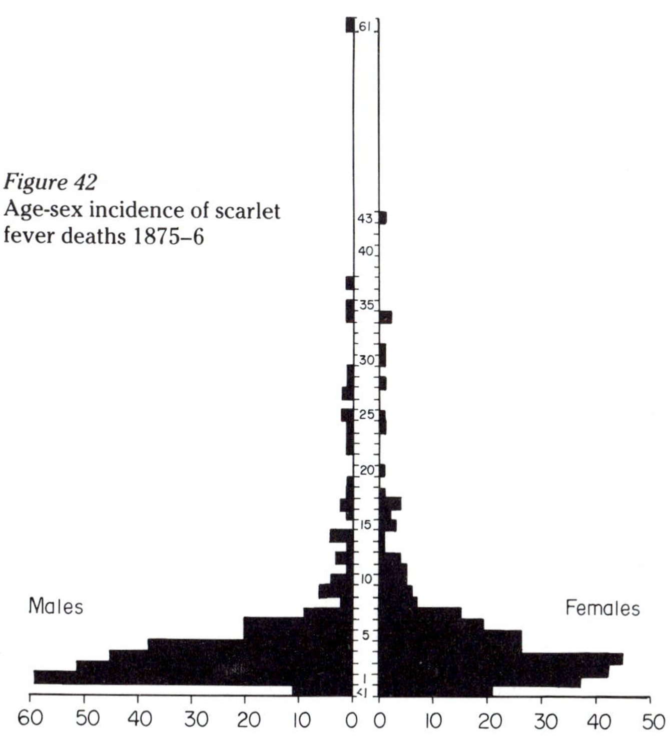

Figure 42
Age-sex incidence of scarlet fever deaths 1875–6

Table 22 Deaths from Scarlet Fever by Age and Sex 1875–6

Age group	*Males*	*Females*	*Total*
0–4	209	171	380
5–9	57	73	130
10–14	13	16	29
15–19	5	10	15
20–24	2	1	3
25–29	3	2	5
30–34	1	3	4
35–39	2	—	2
40–44	—	1	1
45–49	—	—	—
50–54	—	—	—
55–59	—	—	—
60–64	1	—	1
65 +	—	—	—
Not stated	3	2	5
Total	296	279	575

Source: Registrar-General, Death Records, 1875–6.

deaths came from the ranks of the children of the city's clerical workers, owners of business and property and professionals and gentlemen. That this really reflects a widening of the social net of disease is doubtful, however, as between 1867 and 1875–6 there had been increasing differentiation of Sydney's employment structure, particularly in the area of white-collar workers and small businesses.

COMPLICATIONS

Just over one-third of all deaths involved complications in 1875–6, the commonest being convulsions (36) and kidney disease (32), followed by diphtheria (14), bronchitis/pneumonia (12) and a variety of other complaints (Table 24). Acute nephritis occurred in 10 cases with undefined renal and kidney disease in 23 cases.

Table 23 Deaths from Scarlet Fever by Socio-economic Status 1875–6

Socio-economic status[a]	*Number*	%
Unskilled	116	20.2
Semi-skilled	76	13.2
Small tradesmen	189	32.9
Clerical	57	9.9
Small businessmen/proprietors	76	13.2
Professional/gentlemen	20	3.5
Other	3	0.5
Not stated	38	6.6
Total	575	100.0

Source: Registrar-General, Death Records, 1875–6.
[a] If under 16 years, socio-economic status of father.

Table 24 Major Complications, Scarlet Fever Deaths, 1875–6 Epidemic

Complication	*Number*	%
Convulsions	36	19.7
Kidney disease	32	17.5
Diphtheria	14	7.6
Bronchitis/pneumonia/ congestion of lungs	12	6.6
Dropsy	10	5.4
Ulcerated throat	10	5.4
Effusion of brain	9	4.9
Congestion of brain	8	4.4
Debility	6	3.3
Abscesses	6	3.3
Anginosa	6	3.3
Croup	5	2.7
Erysipelas	4	2.2
Other	25	13.7
Total	183	100.0

Source: Registrar-General, Death Records, 1875–6

OFFICIAL REACTION

In many ways the scarlet fever epidemic was a crucial factor in the development of public attitudes towards infectious disease in New South Wales. It was the first real outbreak of infectious disease to excite official concern and generate public unrest. It also coincided with a period of increasing middle-class concern for sanitary reform and helped focus public attention on disease and the living conditions of the urban poor. Moreover, it resulted in a series of preliminary reports on the causes and prevalence of scarlet fever which produced a series of suggestions for the management of infectious disease cases. To this extent, the epidemic represents an important precursor in the development of public health in New South Wales. Some of the suggestions put forward in 1875–6 concerning segregation and quarantine of scarlet fever cases and the fumigation and cleansing of infected houses were to be put to the test five years later during the smallpox epidemic of 1881–2. In 1875–6, however, they remained little more than cautious suggestions and were not put into operation. The epidemic also saw the first tentative search for causes and the medium of transmission, and although the conclusions advanced very much reflected the prevailing concern with clean water, decent lavatories and drains and pure air, they none the less represent the first official efforts to try to explain disease aetiology and transmission. Early in the epidemic a committee of the Sydney City and Suburban Sewage and Health Board redirected its attention from Sydney's general sanitary and health condition to inquire broadly into the prevalence of scarlet fever. Although the committee's report is brief, it followed up a number of multiple cases of the disease and commented upon the general sanitary condition of such homes. Among other things, it contrasted the low death rate from the disease in some northern suburbs with the experience of inner Sydney and concluded that the lack of closely packed houses, lower population densities and purer air all helped explain the difference in health and mortality (Sewage and Health Board, 1876:6).

About the same time as the Board was conducting its inquiries the independent Health Society of New South Wales published a small four-page pamphlet entitled *Hints for the Prevention of Scarlet Fever*. This and the later official government memorandum *Prevention of Scarlet Fever* (May 1876) provide the framework of what was eventually to become official policy in the management of cases of infectious disease in New South Wales. Primarily the Health Society argued for a policy of segregation, quarantine and public cleanliness. Those sick with the disease should be segregated for at least a month and children prevented from attending school. The government memorandum went further and suggested that while no official quarantine law existed, those who were willing should be removed to a well-ventilated detached empty house specifically set aside for the purpose. The Society also suggested ways of neutralizing the poisons of the disease by scrupulous attention to cleanliness within the home and exposure to pure fresh air. The sick should be placed in a large well-ventilated room from which all non-essential items of clothing and furnishing had been removed so as to minimize dirt, which attracts the poison. All rooms within the house should be regularly cleansed with carbolic acid, Condy's fluid and chloride of lime. Bed linen should be changed every day and the soiled linen immersed in a bucket of water and chloride of lime or carbolic acid. During the course of the illness the patient should be twice a day rubbed all over with sweet oil, lard or fat. After the patient had recovered (or died), all bedding and clothing should be thoroughly fumigated by burning sulphur in the closed-up room. In conclusion, the Society added that 'the after effects of scarlatina are sometimes very serious and generally traceable to the suppressed action of the skin; it is therefore important that the convalescent should wear flannel and not be exposed too soon or suddenly to the inclemency of the weather' (Health Society of N.S.W., 1876:4).

The object of the government memorandum was to provide some broad guiding principles for averting or reducing the virulence of scarlet fever outbreaks. After a brief preamble which referred to the virulence of the disease and the high mortality caused by it in Britain, the report speculated on the more predisposing influences which tend to allow the disease to develop in New South Wales (*Prevention of Scarlet Fever*, 1876:1). Five basic influences were seen as important:

1. *Errors in diet* — largely intemperance, gluttony, insufficiency, fasting or a monotonous diet.
2. *Public and personal hygiene* — personal cleanliness, poor ventilation and drainage, accumulation of dirt.
3. *Personal characteristics* such as heredity, immorality, idleness and fatigue.
4. *Environmental exposure* — exposure to the sun.
5. *Specific disease poisons* which were more or less always present in densely settled localities and which would burst forth given favourable circumstances.

The remainder of the report consists of a series of recommendations concerning unpolluted water, proper drains, properly constructed privies and the removal of rubbish, as well as recommendations dealing with isolation, quarantine, fumigation and the treatment of those ill with the disease.

PUBLIC REACTION

Apart from official concern and the particular measures mentioned above the scarlet fever epidemic has left us almost no record of the public's general reaction to the disease. Apart from reprinting the government memorandum and a series of public health measures adopted by the Central Board of Health in Melbourne, the Sydney newspapers hardly mentioned the outbreak. They seemed much more interested in the disease's progress through Melbourne than in the epidemic raging in their own backyard. In addition, it also appears that the manufacturers of popular medicines had yet to grasp the financial possibilities inherent in epidemics of infectious disease and the newspapers carried no advertisements specifically mentioning scarlet fever. Despite all this, there are fleeting glimpses of the reactions of Sydney's lower classes to the onslaught of the epidemic in some of the official reports, such as the Nesbit family of Hopewell Street, Paddington, who abandoned their house after the death of their three children from scarlet fever (Sewage and Health Board, 1876:6), or Mrs Solomon of Bourke Street, Surry Hills, who in only four days in late November lost her three children and a servant girl from the disease. Her husband had died six months earlier from typhoid. Like the Nesbits, Mrs Solomon fled. Others appeared to have been stunned by the ferocity of the disease but regrettably we will never know what thoughts were in their minds or how they reacted.

CONCLUSIONS

The scarlet fever epidemic of 1875–6 was a severe childhood epidemic which lingered on in Sydney for a considerable period of time. With the benefit of hindsight the epidemic appears as a crucial stage in the development of public health in New South Wales. It produced the first official investigation into the origins and transmission of infectious disease, helped focus public attention on disease and the living conditions of the city's poor, and resulted in the first tentative steps being taken towards an official policy regarding the control and management of epidemics of infectious disease.

CHAPTER SIX

'We Don't Want No Smallpox Here'

The Epidemic of 1881–2

Ban the Chinaman! We don't want no smallpox here.
Sydney street cry in June 1881

IN MAY 1881 Sydney was visited by an epidemic of smallpox which threatened to spread suffering and death throughout the community. The disease broke out in lower George Street in the house of a Chinese merchant. The epidemic that followed lasted until mid-February 1882. During this time there were recorded 163 cases of the disease including 41 deaths but many cases went unreported or were wrongly diagnosed.[1] The epidemic caused a degree of suffering and human tragedy out of all proportion to the numbers actually involved. Such was the public perception of smallpox that the epidemic caused a wave of hysteria and panic to sweep across the city the like of which had never been seen before. In this sense the epidemic was the first in Sydney's history to inflame popular opinion and although the morbidity and mortality produced were small, the epidemic's overall social impact was tremendous. The popular newspapers were full of stories and advertisements designed to fan the growing panic. At a public level the outbreak drew attention to the overcrowded and insanitary living conditions of Sydney's poor and produced a feverish campaign of cleaning, scavenging, disinfecting and fumigating of infected premises and their surrounds. Hundreds of people were forcibly quarantined either in their homes, at the Quarantine Station or at the Coast Hospital while others were detained aboard ships on arrival at Sydney. The epidemic also brought to the surface a number of underlying social tensions that

[1] The official report of the epidemic and Cumpston (1914) record only 154 cases and 40 deaths. Careful reconstruction of the epidemic from contemporary accounts and newspapers, however, indicates the higher number.

threatened to disrupt the fabric of Sydney society. A wave of hostility was directed against the Chinese community, neighbour turned against neighbour, pro-vaccinators battled anti-vaccinators, the authorities squabbled amongst themselves as to how best to handle the outbreak, popular medicine confronted scientific medicine and the medical community were divided in their efforts to explain and confront the disaster.

In many ways the smallpox epidemic represents a watershed in Sydney's social history. Among other things it helped lay the foundations of public health administration. A Board of Health, an Infectious Diseases Act, an infectious diseases hospital (The Coast Hospital), the Medical School at Sydney University and a set of practical regulations and guidelines governing quarantine, isolation and the general management of epidemics of infectious disease, all owe their origin to the epidemic. In addition, the outbreak ushered in a period of considerable public health activity in Sydney culminating in the classic epidemiological reports on bubonic plague in the 1900s by J. Ashburton-Thompson. Finally, the smallpox epidemic provides an insight into how people reacted when confronted by the challenge of life and death.

THE EARLY HISTORY OF SMALLPOX IN AUSTRALIA

Outbreaks of smallpox occurred in Australia between 1789 and 1917 on at least fifteen separate occasions, giving rise to case fatality rates of up to 33 per cent (Table 25). Most of these outbreaks were small affairs, rarely involving more than a handful of cases and deaths, as well as being limited in their geographical extent. Within the context of small, isolated colonial towns and cities, however, their impact was often out of all proportion to the numbers actually involved. It also seems likely that the virulence of particular smallpox outbreaks was related to the level of immunity and vaccination that existed within the community. During the 1881–2 epidemic in Sydney, for example, there was a great rush for vaccination, which may help to explain the much lower case-fatality rate during the smallpox outbreak of 1884–5. Generally, however, the number of people seeking protection against smallpox remained small throughout the last forty or fifty years of the nineteenth century (Figure 43).

Without a doubt the most significant outbreaks of smallpox in Australia's history in terms of cases and deaths are the two early epidemics among the Aboriginal population in 1789 and 1829–45 (if indeed the disease was really smallpox) and the outbreak of the milder variety (variola minor) between 1913 and 1917. In terms of community reaction, however, it was the 1881–2 epidemic in Sydney and the two outbreaks in Launceston in 1887 and 1903 that produced the greatest public outcry and caused the most disruption.[2]

Like that of most other infectious diseases the history of smallpox reveals a recurring theme — importation by ship from the Old World, dissemination by close personal contact in the innermost residential areas of the main cities, lack of effective measures of treatment and control, and an initial period of virulence followed by a lull when the disease disappeared, only to be later reintroduced and

[2] See Roe (1976) for a discussion of the Launceston epidemics.

Table 25 Major Smallpox Outbreaks, Australia 1789–1917

Date	*Months*	*Location*	*Cases*	*Deaths*	*Case fatality rate*
1789[a]	Apr.–May?	Sydney/N.S.W.	000's	000's	?
1829–45[a]	?	N.S.W./Victoria	000's	00's	?
1857	Oct.–Nov.	Melbourne	16	4	25.0
1860–9[a]	?	Northern Territory	000's	00's	?
1868–9	Nov.–May	Melbourne	43	10	23.3
1872	July–Aug.	Bendigo	7	0	0
1877–8	Dec.–Jan.	Sydney	12	3	33.3
1881–2	May–Feb.	Sydney	163[b]	41	25.1
1884–5	Aug.–March	Sydney	64[c]	4[c]	6.3
1884–5	Aug.–March	Melbourne	56[c]	6[c]	10.7
1884	July	Border Town	3	0	0
1887	Aug.–Oct.	Launceston	33	11	33.3
1893	Apr.–May	Perth	52	9	17.3
1903	June–Aug.	Launceston	66	19	28.8
1913–17[d]	Apr.–Dec.	Sydney/N.S.W.	2392	4	0.2

Sources: Cumpston, 1914; Dixon, 1962; Director-General of Public Health, Report 1913–17; Tidswell, 1898.
[a] Aboriginal population only, no data available.
[b] Includes 1 case at Bega, 1 case at Lismore and 6 cases from the SS *Garonne*.
[c] Undoubtedly an underestimation of true level of cases and deaths.
[d] Variola minor outbreak.
? Not known.

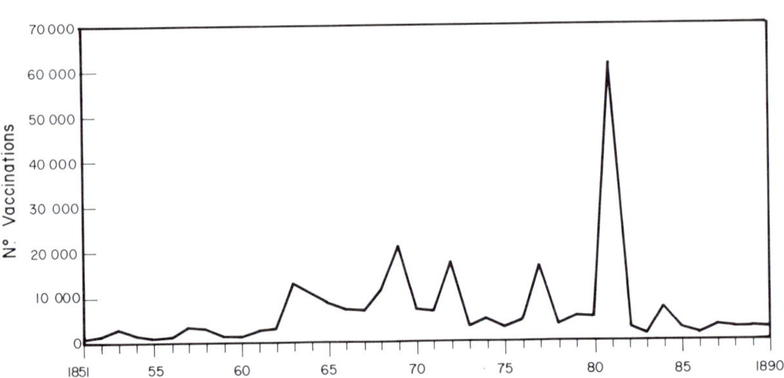

Figure 43 Numbers vaccinated against smallpox in New South Wales 1851–90

recommence the cycle. In this manner Sydney suffered periodic bouts of infectious disease throughout most of the nineteenth century. Between 1820 and 1836 there are scattered references to smallpox cases aboard ships arriving at Sydney but it is not until the 1850s that there seems to have taken place a substantial increase in the number of ships arriving with a record of the disease on the voyage. The twenty or so years after 1881 represent the peak years for the disease in Australia

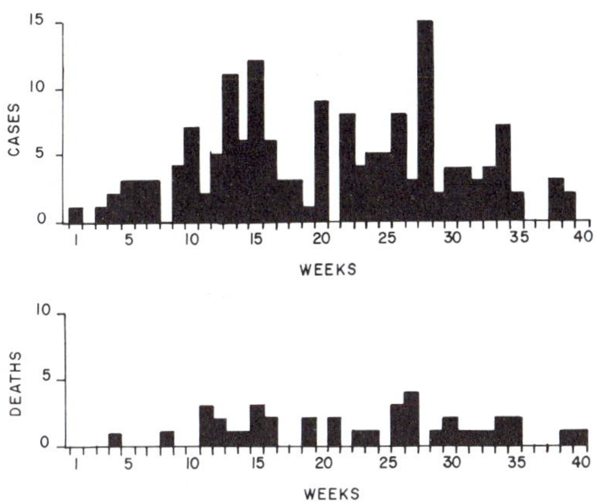

Figure 44 Temporal distribution of smallpox cases and deaths 1881–2

with a total of 437 recorded cases and 90 deaths, not counting cases aboard arriving ships that were quarantined on arrival. It also seems possible that smallpox may have become endemic in Australia in the period 1881–7.

THE 1881–2 EPIDEMIC: TEMPORAL PATTERNS

The first official case of smallpox in Sydney was reported on 25 May 1881 although it was not until some time after that the authorities could agree on a positive diagnosis. The case involved the 17-month-old son of On Chong, one of Sydney's leading Chinese merchants who lived and carried out his business in No. 223 Lower George Street. The source of the child's infection remains obscure although there is some evidence to suggest that he caught the disease from his nurse who apparently had developed a similar eruptive disease approximately two weeks before (see *SMH*, 16 July 1881:16). Where his nurse caught the disease remains a mystery. There is no record of the authorities ever contacting her and consequently the source of the epidemic cannot be effectively traced. Officially smallpox was present in Sydney from 26 May 1881 until 19 February 1882, a total of 271 days during which time 163 cases and 41 deaths were officially notified. Probably there were many more cases, possibly as many as 250, for as the epidemic progressed many people hid their sick away and refused to notify the authorities.

After a slow start the epidemic gathered momentum towards the end of June. As Figure 44 indicates, the overall temporal form of the outbreak approximates an epidemic curve although in this case one with a bimodal distribution with peaks in weeks 13–15 and week 28. Just over 71 per cent of all cases occurred in two major time periods within the epidemic. The first, a ten-week period from late July to late September, produced 59 cases; the second, a nine-week period from early October to the beginning of December, 57 cases. This was followed in late December–early January by a short reprise which was to some extent influenced by the landing of six new cases from the SS *Garonne* which arrived in January 1882. Figure 44 also illustrates the temporal distribution of deaths during the epidemic and although the numbers are small the majority took place within two periods, a six-week period extending from the first week of August to the second week of September and a ten-week period from mid-November to late January. The general form of the epidemic bears all the hallmarks of a contact-transmitted disease and the length of time that it remained in the Sydney community was closely related to the slow smouldering nature of the disease, the length of incubation period, the number of susceptibles and the intimacy of personal contact in high risk areas.

GEOGRAPHICAL DISTRIBUTION

Although the cases of smallpox occurred over a widespread area of the metropolitan area, the full impact of the epidemic fell mainly upon a handful of residential areas located in and near the city centre. Five localities in particular suffered. An area in Sussex Street around Fowler Square, the northeastern tip of Pyrmont, part of lower Woolloomooloo, an area stretching from Macquarie Street South to Surry Hills, and the industrial suburb of Alexandria-Waterloo. The remainder of cases

Table 26 Cases and Deaths by Place of Residence, Smallpox Epidemic 1881–2

Geographical area	*Cases*	*Deaths*	*Case fatality rate*
Fowler Square/Sussex St	33	8	24.2
Pyrmont	30	9	30.0
Woolloomooloo	19	4	21.1
Macquarie St South/Surry Hills	13	3	23.0
Waterloo/Alexandria	13	4	30.8
Haymarket/Ultimo	9	3	33.3
Glebe	7	3	42.3
SS *Garrone*	6	2	33.3
The Rocks/Lower George St	5	1	20.0
Redfern	3	—	—
Woollahra	2	2	100.0
Balmain	2	—	—
Croydon	2	—	—
Camperdown	1	—	—
Moore Park	1	—	—
McDonald Town	1	—	—
Druitt Town	1	—	—
Campbelltown	1	—	—
Field of Mars	1	—	—
Burwood	1	—	—
Quarantine Station	1	—	—
Bega	1	—	—
Lismore	1	—	—
Not stated	9	2	33.3
Total	163	41	25.1

Sources: *SMH*, 1881–2; Board of Health, 1883; Cumpston, 1914.

were scattered about the inner city as illustrated in Figure 45 and Table 26. Together these five areas accounted for 66 per cent of all cases and 68 per cent of all deaths. Largely without exception these areas offered accommodation to many of the city's least affluent and most disadvantaged residents in undistinguished and often depressed tenements and boarding houses. Living and working conditions were severely depressed, with physical decay, overcrowding, communal water and sanitary facilities and contaminated water and food supplies. Poverty, overcrowding and poor sanitation greatly contributed to the spread of the disease.

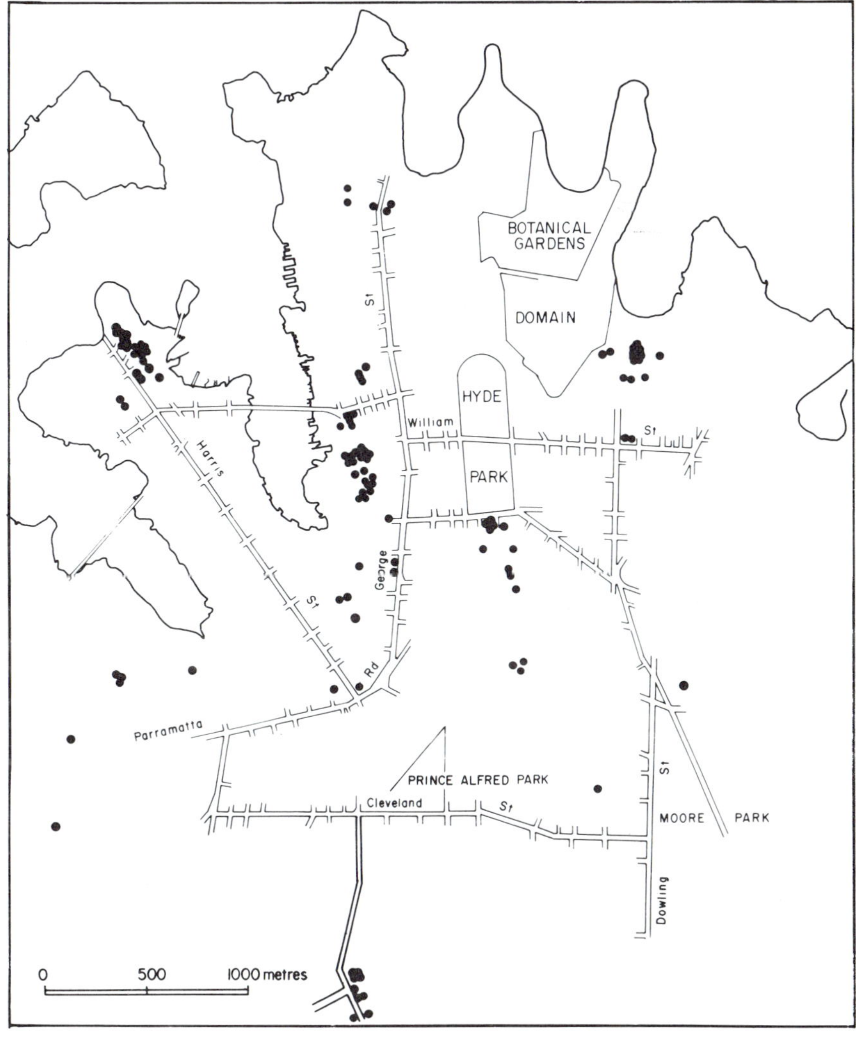

Figure 45 Spatial distribution of smallpox cases, City of Sydney 1881–2

SPATIAL DIFFUSION

Figure 46 graphically illustrates the broad areal expansion of the disease through the inner city of Sydney and traces the interconnections and linkages between the various outbreaks. This diagram also indicates the reasons for the disease's apparent long-distance jumps as in the occurrence of cases at Croydon, Druitt Town, Glebe and Waterloo. In some cases parts of inner Sydney suffered not one but several waves of the disease. As Figure 46 shows, the index or first case can be traced to On Chong's premises, from where the disease spread to Surry Hills, Druitt Town, Waterloo and The Rocks. Of these, only the Surry Hills case led to further spread. The early movement of the disease can be directly attributed to (a) a workman employed on or near On Chong's (the Surry Hills case), (b) a neighbour of On Chong's who moved to Waterloo, and (c) a friend who helped him move (Druitt Town case). The Rocks case was probably related to a business transaction. Of these only the Surry Hills case gave rise to a further expansion when contact between children saw the infection leapfrog the inner suburbs to Croydon. In addition, a workman employed on cleansing and fumigating the infected Surry Hills house carried the infection home with him to Glebe. How the disease reached Fowler Square/Sussex Street remains a mystery. Possibly someone living there had contact with either the Glebe or Surry Hills case. Once established in Fowler Square, however, the disease quickly spread, making its way north and south along Sussex and Clarence Streets as well as invading many of the small courts and lanes in between (Figure 47). By the end of September the first wave of the disease had spent itself in this area. Towards the end of October the disease reappeared, reintroduced by a special constable whose job it had been to keep watch over an infected house in Pyrmont. From his house in Sussex Street South smallpox spread to neighbouring houses and produced an additional nine cases. From Sussex Street the infection was carried to Waterloo, Glebe, Redfern, Ultimo, Woolloomooloo and the Haymarket. From Ultimo the disease spread to Pyrmont where it remained until mid-November working its way through a cluster of small working-class terraces in the vicinity of Cross, Church, Pyrmont, Bowman and John Streets (Figure 48). From here the disease was carried back to Sussex Street as well as further afield to Waterloo. The first Woolloomooloo outbreak (Figures 46 and 49) seems to have been restricted to a family who moved from Fowler Square. No additional cases were added until a new focus appeared three months later in Plunkett Street, possibly introduced from contact with Cowper Wharf where smallpox cases were embarked for the Quarantine Station. This outbreak again seems to have been restricted to the one family and no more cases appeared until 2 December when within four days six cases of smallpox were reported at a dairy at the corner of Plunkett and Forbes Streets. From here the disease quickly spread to neighbouring houses including the Eastern Market Hotel and from there to Duke, Charles and Corfu Streets. In a little over a month this mini-epidemic produced seventeen cases of smallpox.

The Waterloo case of 28 July (Figure 46) provides a good example of the role of visiting relatives and friends in helping spread the disease across the city. The initial case of smallpox occurred in the home of a van driver whose work frequently took him to the Fowler Square/Sussex Street area. From his home the disease was carried to Darlington when his family visited relatives.

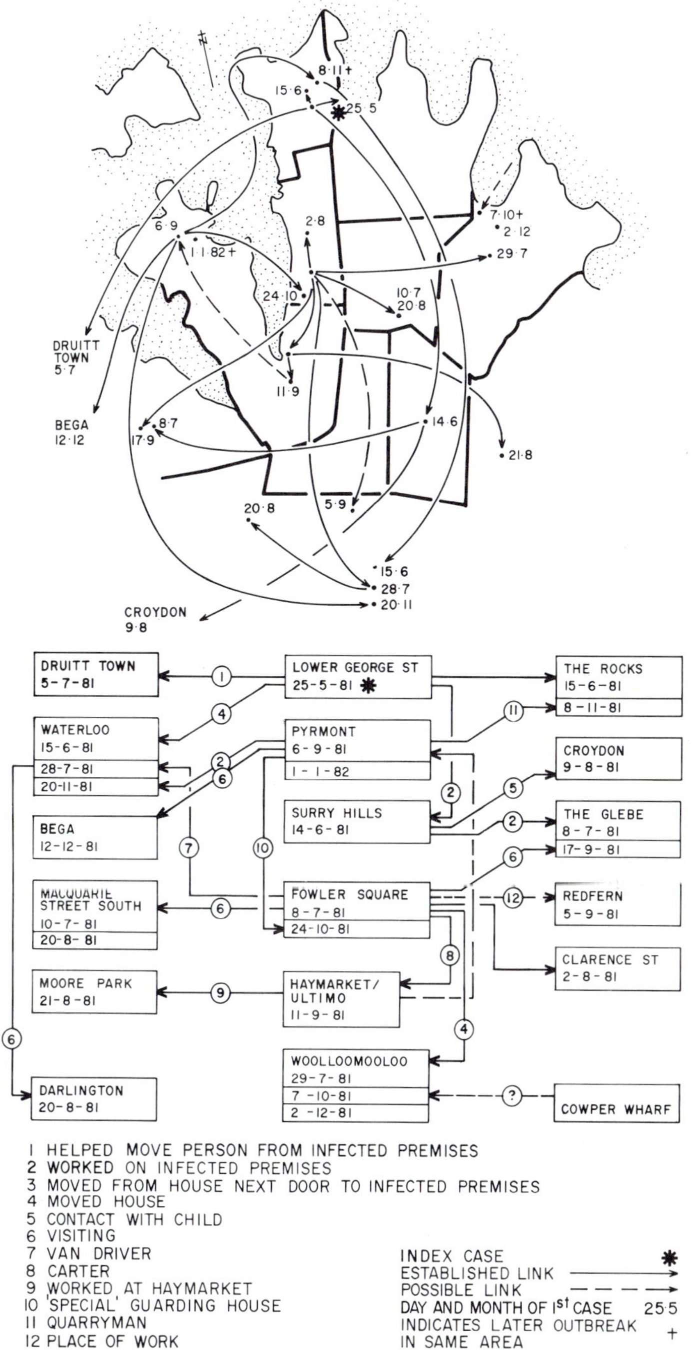

Figure 46 Spatial diffusion and interlinkages, smallpox cases, City of Sydney 1881–2

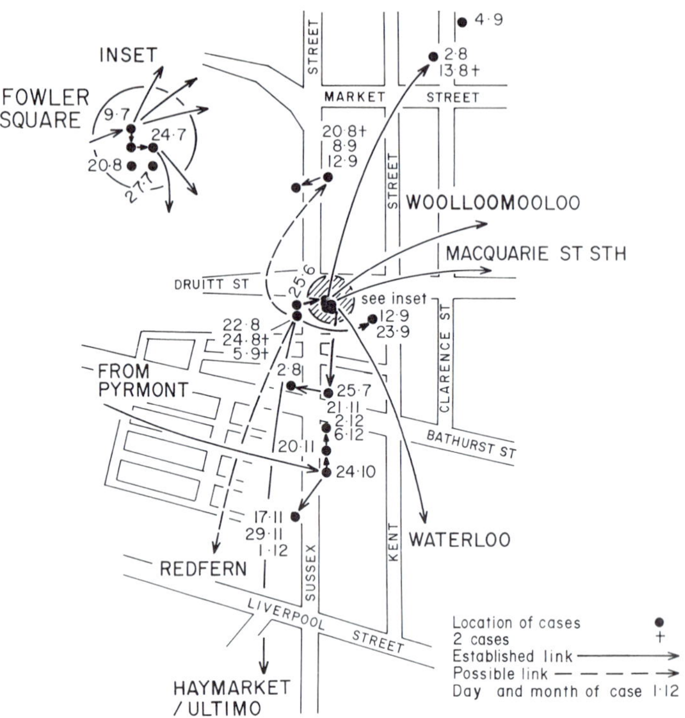

Figure 47 Spatial diffusion, smallpox cases, Fowler Square–Sussex Street 1881

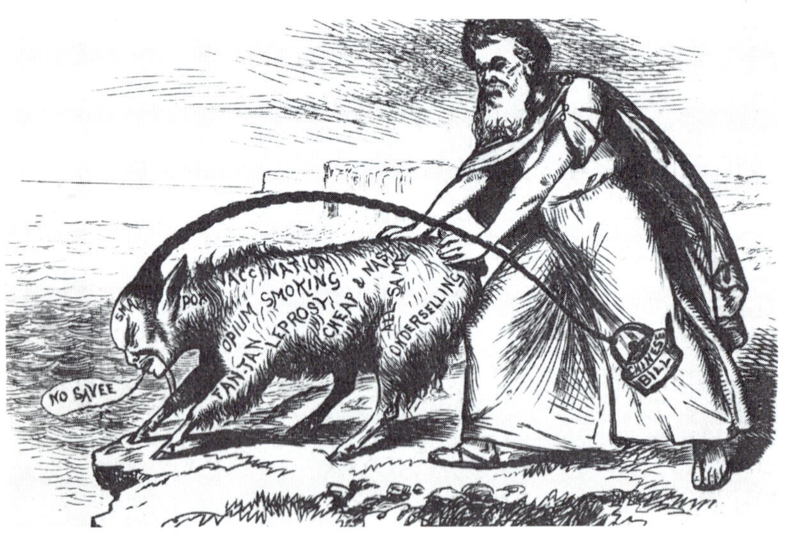

'The Scapegoat'. The smallpox epidemic of 1881–2 became inextricably intertwined with the issue of Chinese immigration and a concentrated campaign of abuse was directed against Sydney's Chinese. Much was made of their apparent susceptibility to diseases such as plague, leprosy and smallpox. Bulletin, *16 July 1881, p. 13. Courtesy the* Bulletin.

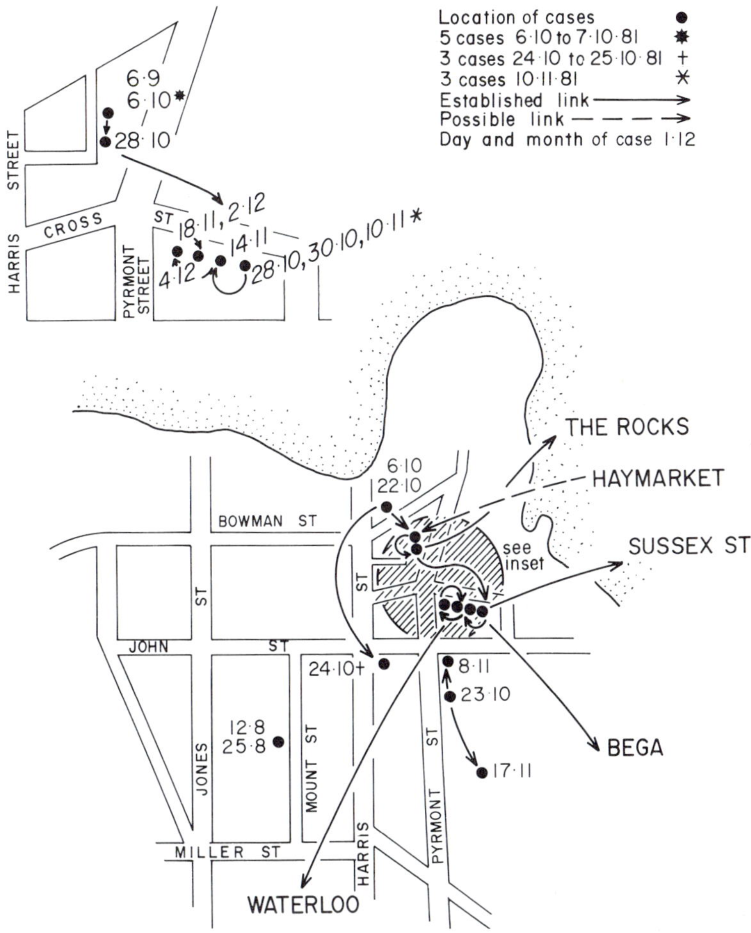

Figure 48 Spatial diffusion, smallpox cases, Pyrmont 1881

Three factors seem critical in understanding how the disease spread across and within Sydney: (1) the spatial mobility of infected individuals and the people in close contact with them; (2) the social and demographic nature of the local community, affecting in particular such things as household size, place of work, place of school, social patterns of visiting, shared facilities; (3) the official measures taken to counter the epidemic, particularly the policy of quarantine, the treatment of infected premises and the policy of vaccination.

THE MEDIUM OF INFECTION

As Table 27 indicates, it is possible in most cases to identify the medium of infection. Five diffusion situations seem important.

1. Intra-household diffusion where the disease spread from one family member to another or to a lodger within the house.

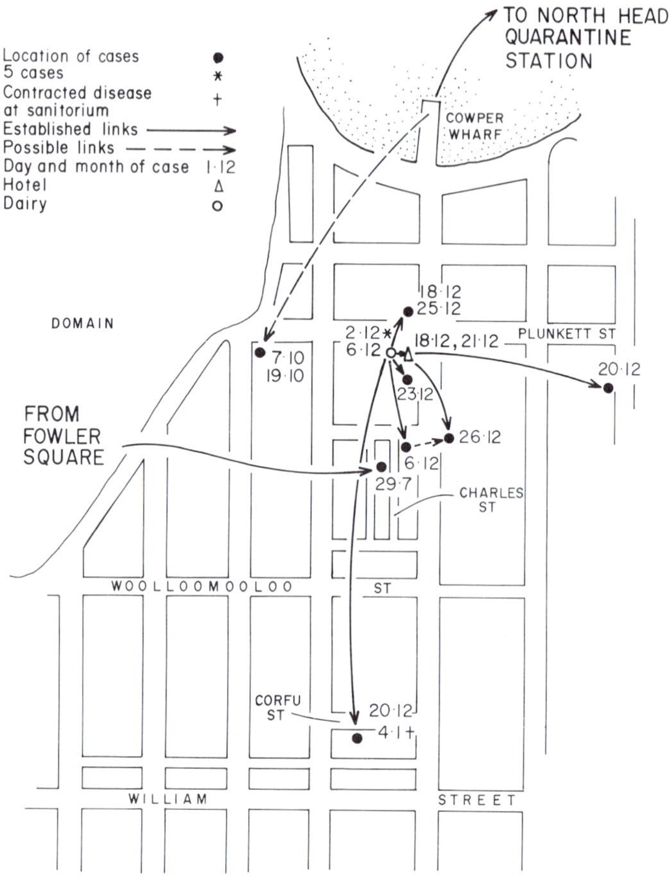

Figure 49 Spatial diffusion, smallpox cases, Woolloomooloo 1881

2. Transfer of the infection from one house to the next-door or neighbouring house largely via patterns of neighbouring and social intercourse (such as the sharing of basic sanitary facilities).

3. Transfer via the medium of longer distance visiting (between kin or friends).

4. Transfer associated with recreation, shopping or work.

5. Where close association with infected persons in quarantine produced the disease.

Together these five situations accounted for almost all the cases of smallpox in Sydney where it has proved possible to identify the medium of infection. Although there were 163 cases reported during the epidemic the number of independent households involved was only 88 (not including six cases on the SS *Garonne* or one grave-digger at the Quarantine Station) and as Table 27 suggests, the majority of cases can be traced directly to intra-household spread (69 cases or 42 per cent). Transfer to a next-door or neighbouring house accounted for an additional 26 cases and visiting relatives or friends another 15.

Table 27 Smallpox, Medium of Infection, 1881–2 Epidemic

	Number of cases	*% of cases*
Intra-household extension	57	35.0
Transfer to next-door house	12	7.4
Transfer to neighbouring house	14	8.8
Visiting	15	9.2
People working near to an infected house	12	7.4
Special constables	3[a]	1.8
Unreported case had previously existed in household	12	7.4
SS *Garonne*	6	3.7
Not traceable	32	19.3
Total	163	100.0

Sources: *SMH*, 1881–2; Board of Health, 1883; Cumpston, 1914.
[a] Includes 1 grave-digger at Quarantine Station.

Table 28 Age-Sex Structure, Smallpox Cases and Deaths 1881–2

	Cases			*Deaths*			*Case fatality rate*		
Age	*Male*	*Female*	*Total*	*Male*	*Female*	*Total*	*Male*	*Female*	*Total*
Under 10	29	27	56	9	8	17	31.3	29.6	30.4
10–20	9	13	22	1	2	3	11.1	15.4	13.6
20–30	19	20	39	5	4	9	26.3	20.0	23.1
30–40	13	8	21	5	1	6	38.5	12.5	28.6
40–50	9	7	16	5	1	6	55.5	14.3	37.5
50 +	1	3	4	—	—	—	—	—	—
Total	83[a]	80[a]	163[a]	25	16	41	30.1	20.0	25.1

Sources: *SMH*, 1881–2, Board of Health, 1883; Cumpston, 1914.
[a] Includes 3 males and 2 females with ages unstated.

DEMOGRAPHIC STRUCTURE

Overall, roughly the same number of males and females caught smallpox during the epidemic, although more males had the misfortune to die from it (Table 28). Sixty-one per cent of all deaths were males whereas they made up only 51 per cent of all cases. In terms of age, the group to suffer the heaviest morbidity and mortality were children aged under 10 years. More than 34 per cent of all smallpox cases and 41 per cent of all deaths were in this youthful age group. The next age group most affected were those aged between 20 and 30 years. In terms of case fatality rates Sydney's middle-aged group (40–50 years) had the highest mortality experience where over a third of all those who caught the disease died. Not far behind were children under 10 years and 30–40-year-olds.

EMPLOYMENT STATUS

The fact that the epidemic occurred mainly in the midst of Sydney's central tenements and working-class residential areas does much to explain why most of those who caught the disease or were in some way touched by it were drawn from the ranks of Sydney's unskilled/semi-skilled and tradesmen classes (Table 29). Most of the tradesmen involved were usually working for themselves and were largely carpenters, butchers, plumbers and the like, some of whom had been employed by the authorities either to repair or demolish infected premises. Only in four cases did the epidemic affect Sydney's merchant or proprietor classes.

THE OFFICIAL REACTION

Despite the fact that Sydney had a history of outbreaks of infectious disease stretching back at least to the 1820s the smallpox epidemic caught the authorities completely by surprise. Certainly there had been nothing quite like it before. Earlier outbreaks of smallpox had largely been restricted to isolated cases aboard arriving ships or as in the epidemic of 1877–8 a handful of cases in the immediate vicinity of the central wharf. Sydney in 1881 was ill-prepared for a major outbreak of a disease like smallpox. There was no administrative or public health structure designed to cope with public health problems, particularly infectious disease. There was no hospital designed specifically to cater for cases of infectious disease and the existing quarantine law applied only to maritime quarantine and the isolation of cases of disease arriving aboard ships rather than to cases of infectious disease arising within the city itself. In addition, there was no formal policy governing the notification of cases of infectious disease or any compulsory vaccination of children. Given such circumstances it is not surprising that official policy was at first *ad hoc*, confused, hesitant and often contradictory. It was not helped in any way by the fact that cases of smallpox continued to be wrongly diagnosed throughout the epidemic. In this respect the city's medical men were hard pressed by the fact that there was a severe outbreak of chickenpox raging at much the

Table 29 Smallpox, Cases and Deaths by Occupational Class (or in the case of wife or child, husband/father's class) 1881–2

	Total	*Male*	*Female*	*Children/ teenagers*
Unskilled	33 (9)	20 (6)	6 (1)	7 (2)
Semi-skilled	10 (2)	5 (1)	3	2 (1)
Skilled (tradesmen)	29 (6)	9 (3)	9 (1)	11 (2)
Small shopkeeper	10 (2)	2 (2)	—	8
Merchant/business proprietor	6	1	3	2
Housewife	11 (1)	—	11 (1)	—
Orchardist	1	—	1	—
SS *Garonne*	6 (2)	3	2 (1)	1 (1)
Not stated	57 (19)	10 (3)	10 (5)	37 (11)
Total	163 (41)	50 (15)	45 (9)	68 (17)

Sources: *SMH*, 1881–2; Board of Health, 1883; Cumpston, 1914.
Deaths shown thus ( ).

same time as the smallpox epidemic in 1881. Many people with chickenpox were diagnosed as having smallpox and sent to quarantine. All this and the many horror stories circulating in the city about the disease, the dangers of vaccination, the conditions at the Quarantine Station, the medical authorities' neglect of people quarantined in their homes and their inability accurately to detect or treat the disease, greatly contributed to the general panic and produced an environment hardly conducive to the orderly or rational management of a major epidemic. Certainly it seems to have produced a situation whereby many people avoided reporting suspected cases for fear of public contempt and possible incarceration at the Quarantine Station.

Throughout the course of the epidemic there was considerable agitation for some sort of compulsory registration of cases of infectious disease, compulsory vaccination and the establishment of a central public health authority. A correspondent to the *Sydney Morning Herald* early in July wrote: '[the] present seasonable alarm of smallpox has contributed to prepare the public mind for recognition of the fact that every citizen has a right to so much protection at the hands of his Government as shall secure him from the grosser evils of foul air, foul water, impure food, unwholesome dwellings . . .' (*SMH*, 8 July 1881).

Throughout the last six months of 1881 the New South Wales branch of the British Medical Association continually lobbied the government on the issue of a central public health authority and the necessity of a notification system for cases of infectious disease. The government eventually responded by appointing a Board of Health consisting of the Mayor of Sydney, the Under-Secretary for the Department of Finance and Trade, the Inspector-General of Police, the Colonial Architect, plus six medical men, one of whom was to be the Health Officer. By mid-July this body had assumed virtual control of the day-to-day running of the epidemic.

To the demands for compulsory vaccination and an act for the registration of cases of infectious disease the government was slow to respond. Despite the establishment of an official Committee of Inquiry into compulsory vaccination in mid-September no decision was reached. By September and until mid-December Sydney was gripped in a vice of growing anxiety bordering at times on panic. There was mounting criticism of the government's handling of the epidemic, particularly of conditions at the Quarantine Station, and of the conflicting diagnoses of competing doctors. This and the increase in the number of smallpox cases towards the end of the year, produced wave after wave of unrest in the city. Finally, in mid-December the government pushed through a bill requiring the compulsory registration of all smallpox cases. It was almost too late as the epidemic was virtually over.

When it came to dealing with the epidemic the authorities were undoubtedly assisted by the fact that the infection had fallen upon sections of the city occupied by Sydney's most disadvantaged groups. This meant that more drastic and ruthless measures could be adopted to prevent contagion and contain the outbreak than if the disease had affected Sydney's more articulate and politically powerful middle and upper classes. In addition, many of the policies tentatively advanced for the control and management of scarlet fever in 1875–6 could now be put into practice with a more ominous disease. Official policy took a variety of forms. In the first place an effort was made to quarantine and isolate all smallpox cases and their immediate contacts. As part of this policy all infected dwellings were barricaded and the public restricted to no closer than 12 feet. Secondly, all infected premises were subjected to a rigorous cleansing, fumigating and scavenging, a policy which was extended to include neighbouring houses and streets. Eventually whole blocks of central Sydney would be virtually closed off as a team of official cleansers and scavengers systematically worked their way from house to house. Thirdly, the authorities offered optional vaccination to all contacts of the disease as well as to the general public. Only in the case of the police force, health workers, cleansing teams, inmates of government institutions and the Chinese was vaccination made compulsory. Finally, there was a series of other measures advanced in an effort to contain the outbreak. These included the closing of several schools and public institutions, the disinfecting of all public conveyances, the establishment of depots for the sale of disinfectants and fumigants and the establishment of an Ambulance and Disinfecting Corps. During the course of the epidemic the resources of the police and health workers were often stretched to the limit. By July it was estimated that one-seventh of the New South Wales police force was employed in quarantine work and the government was forced to recruit a force of special constables to guard infected homes.

QUARANTINE

Early on in the epidemic it was resolved to quarantine and isolate smallpox sufferers and their immediate contacts. The policy, at least in theory, seems to have been that once a case of the disease was suspected then the suspect and his house were placed in quarantine until a time when the disease was either confirmed or otherwise. If the diagnosis proved positive, then all those in the house who were willing were vaccinated, mosquito netting was affixed to all windows, barriers were erected, a police guard was mounted front and back, a yellow flag was hoisted and the neighbours were notified by circular. If the medical officer involved considered the patients fit enough to be removed, and if they were willing to go, they were taken to the Quarantine Station at North Head (later the Coast Hospital). The officer also attempted to persuade the inhabitants of the wisdom of accompanying the patient into quarantine and many seem to have been prevailed upon to accept voluntary exile. Up until the virtual end of the epidemic it seems that formal quarantine at the Quarantine Station or Coast Hospital was not compulsory except in a few cases where it was deemed to be in the community interest to remove the patients. Thus it would appear that the Chinese were rarely offered the choice between staying put or making the trip to formal quarantine.

Quarantine itself took a variety of forms. Those who refused to leave or were too ill to travel were quarantined in their homes. In theory, adequate provision was to be made for their upkeep and nursing, including daily medical visits and the provision of food, medical supplies, bedding and clothes. In practice, however, many of those barricaded at home were virtually ignored and left without adequate care or supplies. The authorities seem to have belatedly recognized such problems by early December when there is evidence that occupants of infected houses who refused to leave were forcibly removed under an order from the government and Executive Council and sent to the sanitorium attached to the Coast Hospital at

Little Bay. Those who elected to go into quarantine were until early December sent to the Quarantine Station at North Head. Later, contacts were sent to the sanitary camp at Little Bay which eventually became the sanitorium attached to the Coast Hospital. By early December all cases of smallpox were under considerable pressure to go to the Coast Hospital and all contacts to the adjacent sanitorium.

Overall almost 900 people were formally quarantined during the epidemic, 163 as cases and the remainder as contacts. An additional 700 or so were detained aboard ships off North Head after their arrival in Sydney. As Table 30 indicates, most elected for quarantine in their own homes. In this they may have been influenced by the many horror stories that circulated through Sydney about conditions and treatment of inmates at North Head. For those sent to the Quarantine Station, removal and leavetaking from home was a highly distressing and chaotic affair. Families were often forced to do for themselves while officials and onlookers kept a safe distance. The removal of Mrs Guildford from her house in The Rocks in July, for example, was watched by approximately two hundred school children recently dismissed from school as well as many others.

In the case of the Chinese, such as Won Ping of Waterloo, formal removal was only accomplished by the police using missiles and long poles. Such were the scenes accompanying removal that the authorities finally decided to remove cases and contacts either in the early hours of the morning or late at night to avoid the possibility of panic and contagion. The police organized the removal of cases and contacts by bus or wagonette from home to the Cowper Wharf in Woolloomooloo, from where the small steam launch *Pinafore* ferried them across to North Head. During this trip cases and contacts were not always segregated, and such was the fear of smallpox that the crew of the *Pinafore* refused to convey cases of the disease aboard their vessel and insisted that they occupy an open boat towed behind. Later on in the epidemic when accommodation at North Head became full, use was made of an old watch-house at the corner of Erskine and Clarence Streets as a temporary holding place for smallpox cases awaiting transfer to North Head.

Once at North Head, cases and contacts, males and females and Chinese were rigorously segregated. All male cases of smallpox (including the Chinese) were placed aboard the *Faraway*, an old barque of 400 tons fitted out as a hospital ship.

Table 30 Smallpox, Cases and Contacts, Place of Quarantine, 1881–2

Place of quarantine	*Cases*	*Contacts*	*Deaths*	*Case fatality rate*
Own home	72	434	22	29.3
Quarantine Station	52	94	14	26.5
Coast Hospital	39	189[a]	5	12.8
Total	163	717[b]	41	25.2

Sources: *SMH*, 1881–2; Board of Health, 1883; Cumpston, 1914.
[a] Includes sanitorium and sanitary camp.
[b] Does not include approximately 380 passengers aboard the SS *Ocean*, 250 on board the RMS *Zealandia* and 100 passengers on the SS *Garonne* quarantined on their respective ships off North Head.

Conditions aboard the *Faraway* were deplorable.[3] The official in charge had no medical training, there were no proper facilities, food and water were scarce and there was a complete lack of nursing and proper medical care. Patients in some cases were left to their own devices to wander on deck at night in their delirium. Conditions at the land station seem to have been considerably better. Here inmates were grouped in three main sections. A series of detached weatherboard pavilions served as accommodation for female cases and convalescents. Female contacts were accommodated in another section while the Chinese occupied a group of tents near the seashore. Wild rumours circulated about conditions at North Head during the first four months of the epidemic. The first contingent of people released from quarantine arrived back in Sydney on Thursday 25 August full of stories of horrible indifference and outrageous neglect. Complaints ranged from coffins being left in full view of patients and contacts, drunken grave-diggers, lack of food and comforts, to women being deprived of their undergarments before being allowed to return to Sydney only half-clad! One man even complained that before he was allowed to leave his watch was dipped in carbolic. Of such volume were the complaints that the government was forced to suspend the Station's superintendent and establish a Royal Commission of Inquiry. Much of the evidence presented represents a damning indictment of the measures adopted for dealing with the epidemic.

As the epidemic progressed it became increasingly clear that the Quarantine Station could not cope with the numbers involved or provide an adequate level of nursing and support care. As early as July the government had appreciated the fact that Sydney needed a fully self-contained isolation hospital located at a safe distance from the city. A site was eventually selected by the Board of Health at Little Bay, 15 kilometres from the city, and it was hoped to complete the hospital within one month. It was not, however, until early December that the new hospital opened its doors to smallpox sufferers. In the intervening period, faced with increasing pressure on accommodation at North Head and growing criticism of living conditions, the government was forced to erect a temporary sanitary camp of tents on the Little Bay site and offer contacts the choice of accommodation here or at home rather than at North Head. On 7 December the Coast Hospital at last was formally proclaimed as a smallpox hospital. Its accommodation consisted of a series of detached pavilions with accommodation for 106 patients, staff residences, a dispensary, store, kitchen, bathroom, laundry and telegraph office. It was staffed by a full complement of medical and nursing staff. The adjacent sanitorium, separated from the hospital by a galvanized iron fence, consisted of five pavilions and associated facilities with accommodation for 42 contacts. By the time the Coast Hospital opened its doors the epidemic had almost run its full course. Only 39 cases of smallpox were treated there although almost 190 contacts were accommodated at the nearby sanitary camp and sanitorium. Conditions at the Coast Hospital/Sanitorium were undoubtedly a considerable improvement on what had been the case at North Head. The *Sydney Morning Herald* records the Christmas Day feast 'of excellent viands [which] caused a large amount of satisfaction' (*SMH*, 27 December 1881:4) and a night or so later 'a very enjoyable evening's enter-

[3] See Gilder (1938) for a brief discussion of the *Faraway* and its role in the epidemic.

tainment, consisting of music, readings, recitations etc. [was] held on Monday pm at the Sanitorium, all inmates taking part' (*SMH*, 28 December 1881:4).

Problems of diagnosis and the general panic plagued the epidemic throughout its course and led to a policy of indiscriminate quarantine of anyone remotely suspected of having the disease or who had somehow come into contact with somebody who had it. A large number of suspected cases and contacts were either sent to quarantine or shut up in their homes on the flimsiest of evidence. Evidence exists of twenty such cases and in all probability the total number may have approached a hundred. In many cases such indiscriminate policy caused considerable personal suffering and tragedy. Two examples illustrate the tragedy of wrongful diagnosis and quarantine. Mrs Bonner was removed to the Quarantine Station as a suspected case of smallpox on 16 July. Her five children aged between thirteen years and eight months were shut up in her house at Ultimo for six weeks and received no visit from the medical authorities during this time. Food was passed through a back window by a friendly neighbour. Mrs Bonner was not released until 17 August even though her symptoms had disappeared three days after her removal. David Forrest of Waverley was sent to quarantine in late July for absolutely no reason other than that he tried to board a bus at Waverley with the greater part of his face concealed by a bandage. He was refused passage on the bus, the police were called and found him to have a slightly disfigured face. Despite this, David Forrest was taken to North Head and spent five weeks in quarantine. After his release he returned to find his business in ruins and himself shunned by neighbours and friends. Dispirited, he pressed the government for compensation but to no avail. Many people suffering from chickenpox were also wrongly diagnosed and sent to the Quarantine Station.

CLEANSING AND SCAVENGING

The second measure adopted by the authorities to contain the epidemic was in line with the belief, strongly stated by municipal and health authorities throughout the nineteenth century, that cleanliness was next to godliness and a formidable antagonist of disease. This was a policy of cleansing, fumigating and scavenging of all infected houses, yards and surrounding streets. After the third case of smallpox on 15 June the Mayor of Sydney dispatched a gang of scavengers to Surry Hills with instructions to cleanse the streets, back lanes and yards in the neighbourhood of the infected premises. Within two days the residential block bounded by Albion, Elizabeth, Foveaux and Riley Streets had been invaded by a team of cleansers and scavengers treating the streets and lanes with carbolic acid, removing rubbish and disinfecting houses, yards and fences. As the epidemic progressed large areas of central Sydney were officially declared infected zones and their streets cordoned off by barriers. A team of official cleansers then moved in and systematically worked from building to building, disinfecting, limewashing, removing rubbish and demolishing dilapidated structures. The Chinese, never well treated at the best of times, had a hard time of it. Their houses and shops were subjected to more drastic measures than the general population. Won Ping's house and outbuildings in Botany Road, Waterloo, for example, were burnt down after the occupants had been forcibly removed. The government also carried out a

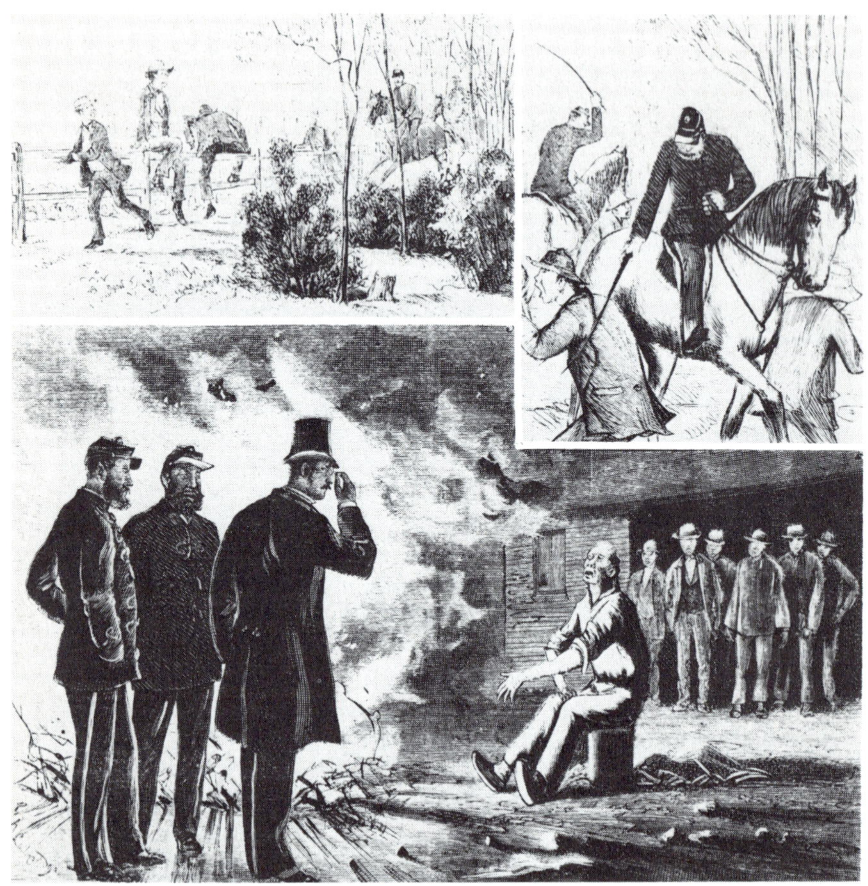

The discovery of a Chinese smallpox patient at Druitt Town. During the epidemic Sydney's Chinese community was subjected to particularly severe treatment. Sydney Mail, *16 July 1881, p. 105. National Library of Australia*

survey of all Chinese dwellings in central Sydney and the newspapers had cause to remark on the degree of overcrowding, lack of ventilation and general filth discovered. By the end of June the Sydney City Council began issuing notices to all householders calling for the removal of all house refuse and indicating depots where disinfectant and fumigants could be purchased.

Early in July the Board of Health recommended the formation of an Ambulance and Disinfecting Corps. Six men under the charge of a senior police constable commenced work late in July charged with cleansing and disinfecting infected houses. Their instructions stated that they should

> cleanse and disinfect a house or building . . . [with] all care . . . that no property is unnecessarily damaged. . . . All clothes, mattrasses, bedding, carpets . . . etc; which may *have come into contact with a patient are to be burnt* upon the premises. Those which have not been in the room with the patient are to be disinfected. . . . All papered walls of every room

which has been occupied by a patient are to be stripped; a hot solution of carbolic acid . . . being used for the purpose. All wall paper to be burnt after removal from the walls. All whitewashed walls, ceilings, etc; to be thoroughly scraped, and the scrapings burnt. All walls . . . to be lime-washed . . .

Yards were also to be thoroughly cleansed and all refuse and rubbish removed. Finally, all rooms were to be sealed by pasting coarse brown paper over the fireplace and window and door joints, and a large tin-iron basin two-thirds filled with water over which a tripod and iron dish of sulphur was to be ignited. The house was to be left like this for at least six hours (Board of Health, 1881–2: Appendix F). By the end of August the Ambulance Corps numbers had to be increased to fourteen and in addition the Sydney City Council continued to employ three carts and three labourers on foot to water the streets with disinfectant as well as sixteen carters and labourers to remove rubbish. The vigour with which these teams carried out their appointed task is attested by the large number of complaints from people returning to their homes from quarantine to discover their furniture broken or badly mistreated, a thick crust of lime over everything, household goods missing and fences and outbuildings knocked down. In October the Ambulance Corps was again expanded to include not only cleansers, labourers and carters but also carpenters, painters, blacksmiths and gardeners and a practical chemist and deodorizer. The activities of the Corps became one of the sights of Sydney and wherever they went they were accompanied by a vast throng of children and local residents.

VACCINATION

In 1803 Governor King requested the dispatch of vaccine matter to New South Wales. After its arrival in 1804 a handful of children in Sydney were vaccinated. In the same year cowpox seems to have become established in the colony and parents were invited to avail themselves of the opportunity of having their children vaccinated. After this an indigenous source of vaccine lymph appears to have died out, to be periodically reintroduced from England. No compulsory vaccination act was ever enacted in New South Wales. There is no record of the number of vaccinations taking place before 1851 and even after this date the available figures do not include those performed by private medical practitioners. Generally the colony exhibited a basic apathy towards smallpox vaccination except in the years when epidemics threatened. Consequently the peaks on Figure 43 correspond closely with the outbreaks of smallpox in Australia. To a large extent the general lack of interest in vaccination was related to three important factors which were to play a major role in the 1881–2 epidemic. Firstly, there was suspicion that vaccination carried with it the threat of inoculating the body with a variety of other diseases such as syphilis and leprosy. Secondly, there was a widely held belief that vaccination was not necessary, given the infrequent and small-scale nature of smallpox outbreaks during the nineteenth century despite a very low number of people vaccinated. Finally, there was the misguided belief that Australia's general isolation and policy of maritime quarantine offered a sure bulwark against the invasion of diseases like smallpox.

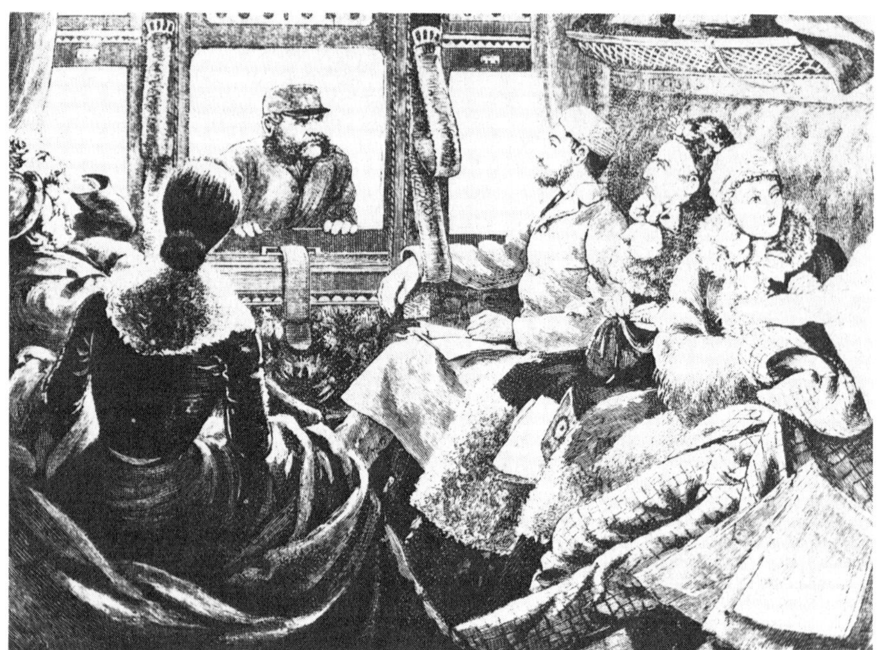

Scene at Albury railway station: 'Any smallpox in this carriage?' Rigorous efforts were made to confine the epidemic to Sydney. Travellers by rail and sea were frequently subjected to quarantine and health checks.
Sydney Mail, *6 August 1881, p. 233. National Library of Australia*

After the second case of smallpox was officially declared in early June 1881, the government issued instructions to vaccinate all police, government boatmen, health workers, ambulance men and cleansers as well as all inmates of public institutions. In addition, it advertised that the public could obtain vaccination at the Town Hall every day. On the next morning a vast crowd assembled outside the Town Hall and more than two hundred had to be turned away after supplies of lymph ran out. Throughout July and August the Sydney newspapers were full of letters arguing the pros and cons of compulsory vaccination. Both pro- and anti-vaccination meetings were held in Sydney and at one an Anti-Vaccination League was proposed. Feelings ran high at such meetings and rumours circulated as to the nature of the lymph being used and that it originated from infected adults and children. Many claimed to have been vaccinated and to have subsequently caught the disease. Where anti- and pro-vaccinators agreed, however, was in respect to Sydney's Chinese population. Both were adamant that all Chinese should be compulsorily vaccinated. Here the government apparently agreed, and whereas vaccination remained largely optional for all contacts the Chinese community seems to have had to submit to compulsory vaccination. Despite adverse publicity the government continued to vaccinate all its official staff and institutional inmates and urged all people living in the vicinity of any smallpox case to submit to vacci-

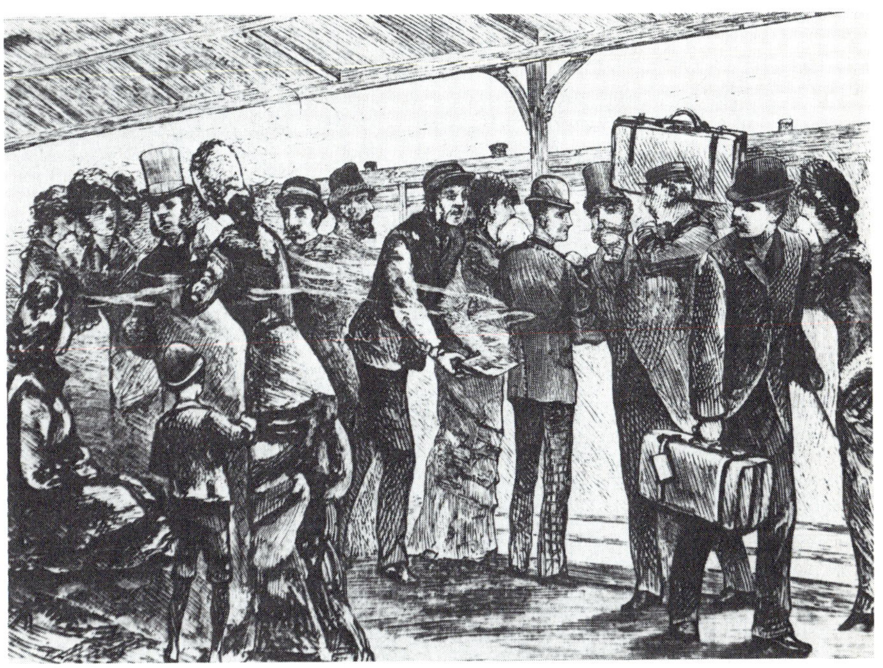

In 1881 efforts were made to fumigate and purify the air to stop harmful miasmas spreading smallpox. Here passengers waiting to board trains on the New South Wales border are being fumigated.
Sydney Mail, *10 December 1881, p. 972. National Library of Australia*

nation. The response to this can be seen in Figure 43. More than 61 000 people came forward, the largest number of any year between 1851 and 1890.

The continuing wrangle between pro- and anti- factions ultimately led to an official inquiry into compulsory vaccination in which most of the colony's leading medical men appeared. The New South Wales cabinet sat for the best part of a week in mid-September as a Committee of Inquiry and verbally examined the principal medical men as to their opinions on vaccination. The proceedings of this inquiry were made public in late October but no definitive statement or conclusions were ever published by the cabinet and no act of parliament ever passed. Fifteen of Sydney's leading doctors gave evidence and all but one strongly supported compulsory vaccination. Only Dr Le Gay Brereton opposed it on the grounds that 'more evils arose from vaccination than from smallpox'. Le Gay Brereton had been one of Sydney's staunchest opponents of vaccination and from early July until late October kept up a veritable flood of letters and articles to all the major Sydney newspapers. He seems to have based most of his opposition on the belief that the increase of smallpox during the nineteenth century was directly related to the increase in vaccination and that vaccination encouraged the emergence of latent diseases as well as introducing new diseases into the body, particularly syphilis. Giving evidence before the Committee he stated: 'I would rather be shot than have anyone of my family vaccinated'. From the cabinet's response to his evidence it would appear that they did not necessarily share his views. Given this and that the weight of medical opinion expressed by the other fourteen doctors was strongly in favour of compulsory vaccination, it is surprising that no positive conclusions were reached. Possibly the cabinet believed that by late September–early October the worst was over and that the problem would solve itself. Possibly they were influenced by the volume of letters that flooded the daily newspapers supporting Le Gay Brereton's views. Whatever the reason, by November public pressure for compulsory vaccination seems to have faded away and its place in the newspaper columns was taken by letters and articles calling for the compulsory registration of all cases of infectious disease.

OTHER MEASURES

In addition to quarantine, cleansing and vaccination the government also employed a variety of other measures designed to restrict the epidemic spreading. Instructions were issued to all asylums and libraries to adopt every possible means to resist the introduction of the disease. In response Randwick Asylum closed its doors to visitors on 16 June and the Benevolent Asylum followed suit a day later. It was also decided that borrowers of books from all public libraries would, if required, have to produce a certificate attesting that they and their families were free of the disease. From late June all Sydney buses and trams were thoroughly cleansed and disinfected every day and notices were issued to all householders in the vicinity of any smallpox case drawing their attention to the need for cleanliness, the location of the closest disinfectant depot and the absolute necessity to report any suspicious illness immediately.

PUBLIC REACTION

Despite the relatively small number of cases and deaths, the epidemic had much in common with classic smallpox outbreaks. It gave birth to a massive upsurge of emotional reaction in the city, at times bordering on mass hysteria and panic. Throughout the epidemic, public reaction manifested itself in a variety of ways, one of the most spectacular and tragic being the search for scapegoats amongst the city's Chinese community.

ANTI-CHINESE FEELING

The origins of anti-Chinese feeling in Sydney and New South Wales lie much deeper than the smallpox epidemic but it did serve to bring long-standing tensions to the surface and recrystallize them in a prolonged outburst of prejudice and violence. Most Chinese in Australia owed their presence to the period immediately following the cessation of transportation when most colonies suffered a severe shortage of labour. In the 1840s and 1850s many Australian squatters saw the

Chinese as a ready source of cheap and reliable labour. An indenture system was soon introduced and by 1850 thousands of Chinese were making the trip to Australia. The discovery of gold in New South Wales and Victoria in the early 1850s radically changed the nature of Chinese immigration. Thousands of Chinese flocked to the diggings, many as ordinary migrants as well as former indentured labourers. By the end of the 1850s there were probably 80 000 Chinese in New South Wales and Victoria alone. Resentment of their presence was not long in coming. Violence and open riots flared between European and Chinese miners during the early 1860s. In 1861, in response to increasing agitation for controls over Chinese immigration the New South Wales government passed the first Chinese Immigration Restriction Act, limiting the number of Chinese that any vessel might bring to New South Wales to one for every 10 tons of cargo as well as providing a poll tax of £10. Later restriction acts increased the ratio of immigrants to tonnage to 1:100.

Throughout most of the nineteenth century anti-Chinese resentment centred on four major issues:

1. Concern about Chinese living conditions, particularly overcrowding, lack of sanitary facilities and filth.
2. Concern over Chinese impact on wage rates and jobs.
3. Concern over Chinese racial distinctiveness and residential exclusiveness.
4. Fear of disease: the belief that the Chinese were much more susceptible to diseases such as smallpox, leprosy and plague largely because of their inherent racial characteristics and living conditions.

In many ways the smallpox epidemic served to highlight these issues and channel public opinion against Sydney's Chinese community. The epidemic seems to have provided the authorities and a number of notable politicians with a handy stick with which to beat the Chinese community. It certainly provided a sure way of mobilizing public opinion into accepting an end to Chinese immigration. Considerable publicity was given to the fact that On Chong's child was the first case, the implication being that the disease had somehow arrived aboard a ship carrying Chinese immigrants. Not until months later was it revealed that On Chong's son may not have been the first case, but such a disclosure received very little publicity. An editorial in the *Sydney Morning Herald* in mid-June, while accepting that 'as a rule coloured races are most susceptible [to smallpox]' (*SMH*, 17 June 1881:4), went on to argue that the disease could just as easily have been brought to Sydney from London as Canton. But such comments fell on deaf ears. Over the next few weeks the papers were deluged with letters calling for an end to all Chinese immigration, their compulsory vaccination and a compulsory 21 days' quarantine for all arriving Asian immigrants.

The government quickly moved to declare China and all its ports infected places and moved to quarantine all ships arriving from Chinese ports. The twelve occupants of On Chong's residence were all vaccinated, against their wishes, and removed to the Quarantine Station. A few weeks later Won Ping's house at Waterloo was razed to the ground. By the end of June wild rumours about the numbers of Chinese with smallpox were circulating in Sydney and the police were kept busy following up countless calls reporting Chinese hiding suspected cases.

People began to boycott Chinese goods and services and the Chinese themselves were often refused entry to trams, ejected from shops and spat at in the streets with the cry 'we don't want no smallpox here!' Fearing the disease and loss of business the merchants and residents near On Chong's place in Lower George Street pressed the government to remove all Chinese from the area and fumigate their homes. On 6 July in his monthly report the medical officer of the Sydney Council referred in derogatory terms to 'the Mongolian case at Waterloo'. By early July the police and public health authorities were hard pressed to handle the volume of complaints about Sydney's Chinese community. The majority of such complaints proved to be completely unfounded, such as the 'dreadful groans' coming from a Chinese house investigated by Dr Hodson which turned out to be a Chinese man snoring (*SMH*, 22 June 1881:6), or the case of the Chinese man seen at the window of a house with his face all muffled up. All the occupants of both houses were dispatched to the Quarantine Station despite the fact that no signs of smallpox were present. The SS *Ocean*, which arrived in Sydney from Hong Kong via Brisbane in late June with upwards of 380 passengers (many of whom were Chinese) on board, was immediately quarantined. Four days later the ship let off its distress guns, having run out of food and water. No sickness was ever reported aboard the ship but it remained in quarantine until late July and on release all passengers had their personal property confiscated and burnt, were stripped naked on the beach, and in exchange for the loss of their clothes each was given one suit of clothes and a blanket.

There seems little doubt that the quarantine laws were utilized to inflame popular passions against the Chinese community. An editorial in the *Sydney Morning Herald* on 30 July saw the situation for what it really was and appealed for calm and moderation in dealing with the Chinese, claiming that the smallpox scare was being aggravated by the Chinese scare. It went on to say that the question of Chinese immigration would soon have to be disposed of and argued against using the quarantine laws as a way of preventing Chinese immigration (*SMH*, 30 July 1881:4). It was too late. Not only were the Chinese increasingly subjected to violence in the streets and their property vandalized but they were also repeatedly attacked on the public platform where a number of politicians made capital by holding them up to public odium and scorn. A new Chinese Restriction Bill was read for the first time in the New South Wales Parliament on 7 July. One of its provisions was to restrict the immigration of Chinese and subject all ships with Chinese passengers, whether smallpox was known to be aboard or not, to a certain period of quarantine on arrival. It was in the emotional environment of disclosures of new smallpox cases every day and the rising tide of anti-Chinese feeling that the bill was debated. By the time the bill reached its third reading at the beginning of August anti-Chinese feeling in Sydney was at fever pitch, despite the fact that there had been only three Chinese cases of smallpox. Clearly most people held the Chinese community, and On Chong and Won Ping in particular, responsible for the outbreak. By the end of August the bill had passed the Legislative Council and received royal assent. Three weeks earlier the residents of Waterloo had met to form a committee to raise money for a presentation to the child Lily Goldfinch who first informed the police on Won Ping.

IN QUARANTINE
S.S. OCEAN
400 PASSENGERS
NO WATER
NO SICKNESS ON BOARD
I'll send someone to give them the Small— I mean the necessaries required.
The man he sent.
What a name I shall make! 400 cases of Small Pox!! Then for my Chinese Bill!!!
H. HUNT
But they declined the proffered aid
And suffered in consequence
IN QUARANTINE
This comes of talking to that d— bobby whom I sent on board the 'Ocean'

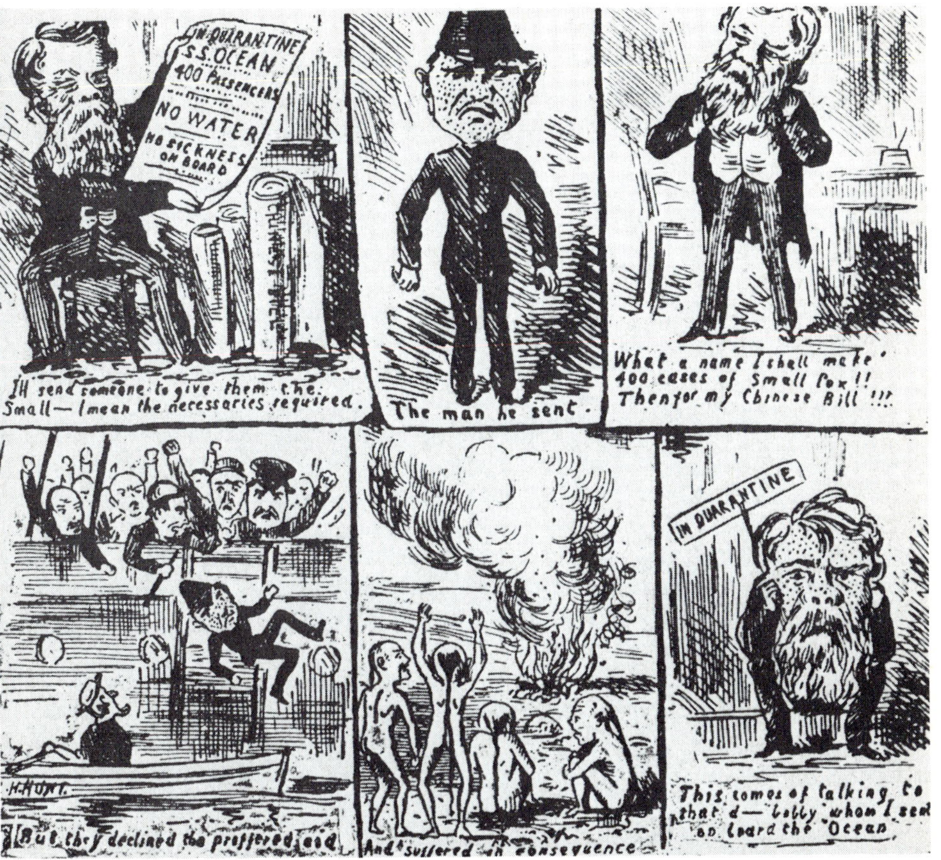

'Parkes and Pustules'. How the *Bulletin* summed up the events surrounding the quarantining of the SS *Ocean* and more than 380 passengers in 1881.
Bulletin, *6 August 1881, p. 4. Courtesy the* Bulletin

PANIC AND HYSTERIA

By August, Sydney was in the grip of mounting fear and terror as wave after wave of panic swept the city. Largely the panic stemmed from dread of the disease and fear of contact with those who had contracted it, the indiscriminate policy of quarantine and the general rumours circulating about vaccination, the Chinese and cleansing. The newspapers did much to fan the growing unease by regularly printing stories of 'The Great Plague' and 'The Black Death' as well as graphic descriptions of the symptoms of smallpox and the names and addresses of recent cases. Sydney's medical men pontificated at endless public meetings, produced countless reports and pamphlets and generally argued amongst themselves over the diagnosis and treatment of particular cases. Panic and hysteria manifested themselves in a variety of ways. The outpouring of violence and discrimination against the Chinese community has already been mentioned. Another example was the mass incidence of spying and reporting on neighbours. During October and early November the Board of Health and the police received dozens of letters informing on people suspected of having smallpox or acting suspicously. Most were simply malicious, reporting anything from simple cases of measles, chicken-pox, pimples or indigestion. The sad thing about many of these cases, however, is that despite the accusations proving unfounded many of the people involved still ended up at the Quarantine Station. The case of David Forrest has already been mentioned but he was only one of many. Possibly as many as a hundred people were sent to the Quarantine Station or incarcerated at home without valid reason. Some of these people had the misfortune to catch smallpox while in quarantine. One such was the child of John Hughes, whose only mistake was to live close to On Chong and who was quarantined on 16 June for five weeks. The child died from smallpox at North Head at the end of June.

The shortcomings of the authorities began by mid-August to excite angry comment. When the first detachment of people released from quarantine arrived back in town late in August some, such as the Keats family of Cumberland Street who had owned a boarding house from where a smallpox case had been removed, had been in quarantine for more than ten weeks without showing any evidence of the disease. On their return they found their boarding house badly damaged by the official cleansing teams. All returnees were unanimous in their criticism of conditions at North Head and their manner of removal and subsequent treatment. Complaints and horror stories about quarantine continued to circulate until the end of September as more and more people were returned from quarantine, many to discover their homes and contents in a shambles or at best encrusted by a thick coating of lime. In September rumours swept the city that the government was about to pass a bill giving it power to possess any infected home and put a match to it. The prospect of enforced quarantine obviously did not appeal to everybody, particularly given the stories circulating about conditions at North Head. Equally disturbing were the reports of people locked up in their own homes and left to their own devices. The end result was that people undoubtedly avoided reporting suspected cases within their own families because of fear of either quarantine or loss of business. In October a mob of local residents, infuriated that the Board of Health had delayed demolishing a dilapidated terrace in Glebe from where a smallpox case had been removed, took the law into their own hands and knocked the house down and removed all the building materials.

Panic and uncertainty also surrounded vaccination and the debate in the press did little to alleviate matters. Many declined to be vaccinated unless they were given an assurance that the matter had been taken from a calf or infant. Throughout the epidemic there was considerable diversity of opinion as to the reasons for the spread of the disease and the remedial measures that should be advanced to combat it. Some argued that it was spread by domestic pets, others by the prevailing winds and still others by bank notes passing from hand to hand. The claim that dogs were responsible for spreading the disease in the vicinity of Fowler Square led to dozens of animals being destroyed. The purveyors of disinfectants, purifiers and popular medicines and tonics had a field day. Their products were

Coming up to the Scratch
An infected Goat — Quarantine him!!!
N CHONG
& Co
MERCHANTS
I begin to think that I've got it"
" Out you go John, you and your Small Pox
SMALL POX
C.H.HUNT.
Here comes a Patient!!!
Well my man, what's the matter with you?— S-Small Pox.

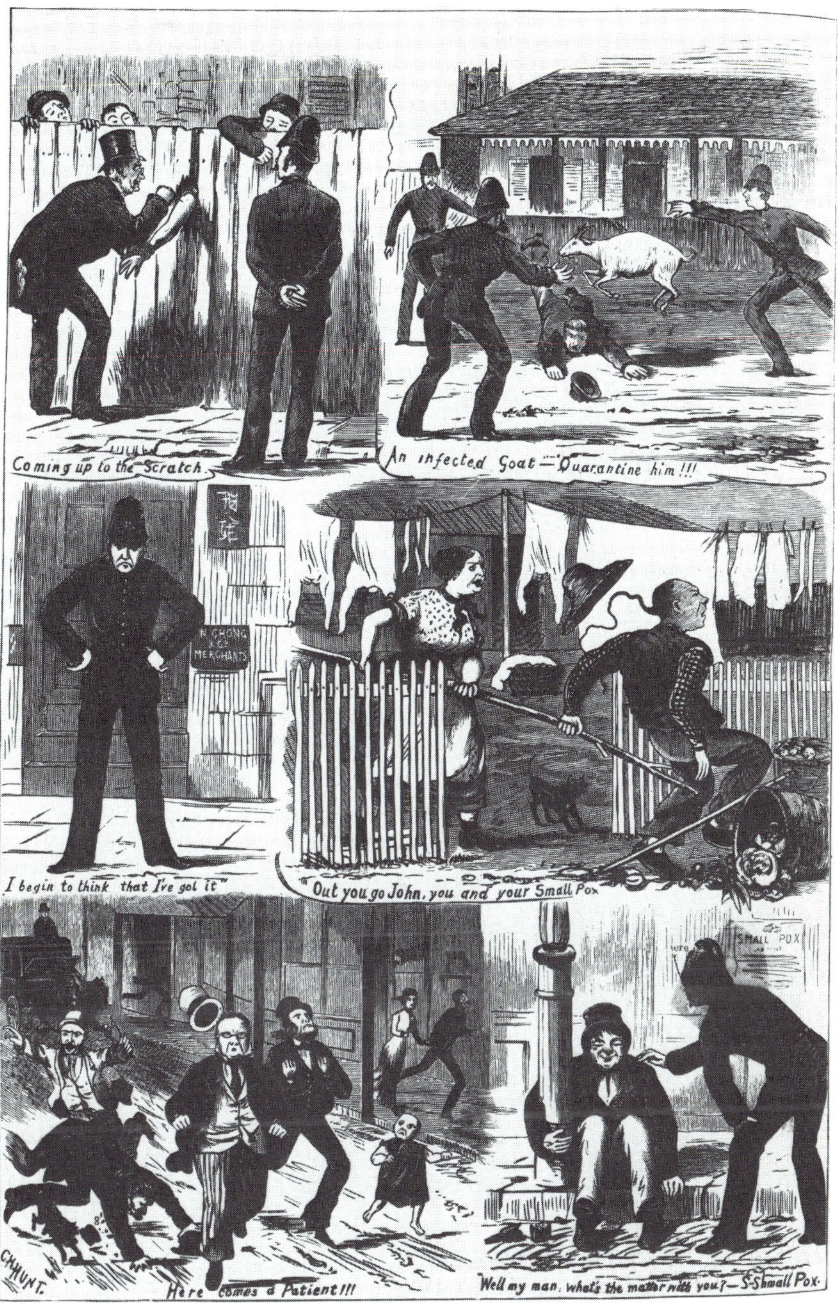

A summary view of the smallpox epidemic in Sydney in 1881–2. Illustrated Sydney News, *9 July 1881, p. 12. From the original in the General Reference Library, State Library of New South Wales*

much in demand. The newspapers were full of advertisements for such products as Bladon's Health Saline or Life Salt, Jeyes Purifier, or Tincture Sulphur, all canvassed as sure preventatives of smallpox. The origin and manner of spread attracted much public comment. A correspondent in the *Sydney Morning Herald* wrote: 'there seems to be some peculiarity in the atmosphere which renders a large population of the citizens susceptible to diseases of the smallpox type' (*SMH*, 26 June 1881:5). It was, however, recognized fairly early in the epidemic that the disease could be traced to one index case, although the actual means of transmission thereafter remained a mystery. At the Sydney Municipal Council meeting of 6 July 1881 the city health officer stated:

> During the past month smallpox has appeared in different parts of the city and suburbs and its spring up in localities so wide apart might cause fear that it has taken a firm footing, but almost for a certainty these cases can be traced to . . . one centre situated in George Street North. Mr. Rout was working on the opposite side of the street and the Hughes family, living in the same direction, both [were] exposed to any germs that might have been carried by the West winds; [the] Guildford family residing in Cumberland Street [were] exposed to infection through East winds. (reported in *SMH*, 7 June 1881:6)

During the epidemic the authorities placed most emphasis on cleanliness, sanitation, decency and order. The belief was that such epidemics would continue as long as filth and bad housing were allowed to continue. Most infected houses and yards were treated with a variety of disinfectants including carbolic acid and chlorine of lime. One of Sydney's leading doctors, J. McCrearie, continued to argue the case for vinegar as a deodorizer and disinfectant. In a letter to the *Sydney Morning Herald* in late August he suggested that people should take ½ oz. of mint sauce with 6 oz. of good mutton or beef and also leave open containers of vinegar around the house. It is somewhat doubtful whether many of the poorer inhabitants of central Sydney would have had access to supplies of good mutton or beef.

The alarm generated by the epidemic spread well beyond Sydney. Panic even took root in New Zealand and from the end of June New Zealand ships were refusing to approach the Sydney wharves and embark passengers and cargo. By mid-July the Victorian health authorities were insisting that all shipping arrivals from New South Wales first stop at Port Phillip Heads for a rigorous health inspection before being allowed to proceed.

CONCLUSION

The last case of smallpox was reported on 19 February 1882 and the last death a week later. All the other Australian colonies and New Zealand were duly notified and Sydney was at last declared a clean port. Early in February the *Sydney Morning Herald* had written in an editorial:

> The wonder is, not that the colonies are being threatened with smallpox, but that they have escaped it so long. . . . considerable doubt exists whether the disease [was] brought here by the Chinese. . . . we have far more to fear from our own countrymen than from the Chinese. . . . the Government must be held to have blundered a good deal at first — learned wisdom as they went on. (*SMH*, 2 February 1882:4)

Whether this wisdom would be applied to later epidemics remained to be seen.

The matter of compensation remained unresolved, however, and served to keep the epidemic in the public's view for many months. On Chong and Company estimated their losses due to quarantine at £2000 and sent a bill to the Colonial Secretary late in August. By mid-October claims were flooding in and were apparently being dealt with very slowly by Treasury. By December most claims were still outstanding.

CHAPTER SEVEN

The Asiatic Flu

The Pandemic of 1890–1

THE AUTUMN OF 1890 was memorable in Sydney for having witnessed the return in epidemic form, after an interval of 30 years, of the historic disease known as influenza — a disease not normally recognized as being very fatal but one noted as causing considerable discomfort and disablement to a large proportion of the population. As the epidemic was the first major outbreak of influenza since 1860 and the first since the establishment of the Board of Health in 1881 the occasion was deemed important enough to call for an official inquiry and a series of detailed reports into the behaviour and causes of the disease. To this end the chief medical officer, J. Ashburton-Thompson, undertook an extensive questionnaire survey of the colony's medical practitioners in 1890 and 1891, the results of which were published in two voluminous reports.

Asiatic influenza earned its geographical epithet because the pandemic was thought to have originated in Asiatic Russia and entered Europe via Siberia. The pandemic of 1889–92, which affected Sydney in two waves in 1890 and 1891, was the beginning of a new chapter in the continent's epidemiological history. It was the first time Sydney had been caught up in a major pandemic of infectious disease, the earlier pandemics of influenza in 1836–8, 1847 and 1850 being relatively minor affairs. Over the next 30 years Sydney was to be swept up in a number of pandemics leading to the most destructive epidemic of modern times in 1919 when influenza carried off more than 6000 of the city's population and affected at least 290 000 others (Director-General of Public Health, 1920).

THE SPREAD OF THE PANDEMIC

There is conflicting evidence as to the origin of the pandemic but it seems likely that it first appeared in Bokhara in Russia about May 1889 and from there travelled to Siberia where it caused an outbreak in October.[1] From there the disease invaded

[1] The origin and progress of the 1889–92 pandemic is described by Parsons in a series of reports to the Local Government Board in 1891–2; see Parsons, 1970.

European Russia and by the end of December most of Europe was affected. By December the disease had reached London and by February of 1890 had penetrated to north and northwest England. North America was also invaded in December and South America between February and April. The epidemic of 1889–90 seems to have spent itself in Europe by the end of March 1890 whereafter the accent shifted to the southern hemisphere where India, Australia, Southeast Asia and New Zealand were all attacked between February and March. The disease reached Sydney in March 1890 and remained epidemic for some months. About May it seems to have subsided, somewhat later in country districts. Throughout the rest of the year and into the beginning of 1891 there was a number of scattered cases which seems to suggest a continual smouldering of the disease and that the outbreak in 1891 was a recrudescence of the 1890 epidemic rather than a reimportation. Interestingly, in 1890 the disease first appeared in Sydney and from there spread to surrounding rural areas, whereas in 1891 it first appeared in country areas and from there invaded the city.

In the spring of 1891 another epidemic of influenza appeared in Britain, severer and more fatal than that of the previous year. It seems to have first appeared in the towns of Yorkshire but by May had reappeared in North America, Europe and Russia. In September and October there was a severe outbreak of the disease in Australia. From Australia the disease spread to New Zealand and from there to many of the Pacific islands. Unlike the earlier outbreaks of the disease the 1891 epidemic spread with great rapidity and caused high mortality. Whereas the 1890 outbreak had resulted in only 4523 deaths in England and Wales, the 1891 outbreak claimed about four times this number and in parts of Europe the disease had an incidence of 40–50 per cent and a mortality rate of 0.5–1.2 per cent (Parsons, 1970). In Sydney, as in the rest of Australia, the second wave of the epidemic in 1891 was far more serious than the first and caused many more deaths. In 1891 the epidemic was responsible for 234 deaths but possibly 100 000 people or more caught the disease. To this extent the epidemic had more in common with the twentieth than the nineteenth century in so far as it produced an extremely high morbidity (i.e. number of cases) but a relatively low mortality.

'SHEARING SHED' OR 'FOG' FEVER — A FORERUNNER?

One interesting sidelight to the epidemic was the speculation surrounding the origin of the disease and its means of transmission. In 1891 some debate took place as to whether the epidemic was an extension of an influenza-like illness highly prevalent in New South Wales rural areas in the years prior to 1890.

In 1885 a highly contagious disease similar to epidemic influenza suddenly appeared throughout parts of New South Wales and Victoria. Mainly concentrated in rural areas the disease appeared to be closely associated with the crowding of men and animals in sheds during the shearing season. The disease went under a variety of local names such as 'shearing shed fever', or 'fog fever' in Victoria (after a season of particularly severe fogs). In New South Wales it was also referred to as 'Temora rot', 'shearer's catarrh' and 'dog disease', the latter apparently because of the amount of discharge from nose and eyes associated with the disease. The disease spread from shearing sheds to invade the surrounding population, particularly in small country towns. The symptoms of the disease were dryness and soreness of the nose and pharynx followed by prostration, chills, pains in the limbs, headache, fever and general malaise, with temperatures in the range of 39–40.5°C. The illness usually lasted for approximately three to four days with rapid recovery, although relapses were common. In many cases complications such as pneumonia and bronchitis were recorded. Contemporary observers noticed that the disease seemed to be more prevalent during the spring when men became easily overheated working in the sheds and when there was a substantial daily range in the temperature regime. One explanation advanced at the time was that the infection was brought on by chills closely related to the activity pattern in the shearing sheds. It was noticed that most shearers perspired freely while working, only to cool down rapidly during meal breaks and smokos. At the time of the 1890–1 influenza outbreak it was widely canvassed that perhaps the disease originated from within Australia and was a particularly virulent form of 'shearing shed fever'. More likely, however, was the fact that this was a form of epidemic catarrh/cold long associated with the peculiarly crowded and unhygienic working conditions connected with shearing. Old sheep-farmers in fact recognized the disease as occurring for many years previous to 1885.

THE DISEASE

In the disease of 1891 the onset of influenza was sudden, usually early in the morning. The incubation period seems to have been about two days with a range of one to seven days. The most common symptoms were headache, pain behind the eyeballs, chills or fever, and a general feeling of malaise. Within a few hours the temperature rose to 39°C or more and many patients were troubled by a short dry cough. The tongue was thickly coated and most suffered muscular ache, particularly in the back, legs and joints. Children often suffered attacks of vomiting and diarrhoea. The fever lasted from approximately three to five days but in many cases the cough, lassitude and general depression persisted for much longer. The disease was primarily a respiratory disease with the virus mostly affecting the cells lining the nose, throat, trachea and lungs. In many cases, particularly among the elderly, pneumonia and bronchitis developed commonly as a secondary bacterial infection. After recovery there was a general feeling of lethargy, weariness and an inability to undertake active bodily or mental work. In severe cases there were ear abscesses, croup and laryngitis as well as pneumonia, pleurisy and bronchitis.

TEMPORAL DISTRIBUTION

Although the first death did not occur until 30 September, the epidemic in Sydney most probably began early in September and was all over by the middle of December. While no record of cases survives, it is possible to infer the overall morbidity pattern from material showing the number of cases among the city's institutional population (see Figure 50). The shape of this epidemic curve merely represents graphically what is obvious for most epidemics of infectious disease, the slow onset followed by the rapidity of spread and the high proportion of individuals attacked.

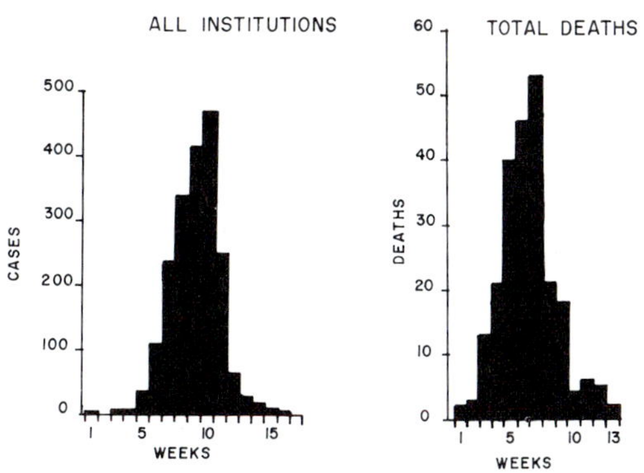

Figure 50 Temporal distribution of influenza cases and deaths, Sydney institutions 1891

By the sixth week (the second week of October) it was apparent that a major epidemic was under way. From 36 cases during the first week of October the numbers leapt to more than 100 in the following week and then increased by more than 100 every week until reaching a peak at the beginning of November when there were 468 cases. After the middle of November there was a rapid decline and by the end of that month the number of new cases per week was down to fewer than 30. Most of the cases occurred in the five weeks between mid-October and mid-November and the peak was reached in a two-week period between 28 October and 10 November when 44 per cent of all cases in Sydney's institutions occurred. By early December it was clear that the epidemic had passed. The pattern of epidemic deaths shows much the same sort of temporal distribution (Figure 50) although the take-off and peak phases were a week or so later, which would seem perfectly explicable given that the majority of deaths were from complications following an attack of influenza.

With respect to the spatial pattern of onset of the epidemic there is little detailed information apart from the data relating to the experience of Sydney's major institutions (Table 31). The Parramatta Gaol and the metropolitan police force exhibited the earliest onset of influenza cases. In both institutions the first case took place in the first week of September (Figure 51). There was then a lull of almost three weeks before cases appeared in the Sydney Hospital. In the following week (30 September–6 October) cases were reported in a number of institutions scattered throughout the metropolitan area. The last of Sydney's institutions to experience the epidemic were the Benevolent Asylum and the Ashfield Infants Home. The temporal distribution of particular institutions is shown in Figure 51.

In some cases the epidemic in these institutions was sharp and short-lived. In the Newington Asylum, for example, the epidemic lasted only four weeks, at Rydalmere Hospital five weeks and at Gladesville Asylum only six weeks (Figure 51). In some institutions it arrived early and persisted until late, as in the case of the metropolitan police force, Parramatta Gaol and St Vincent's Hospital. In others, it appeared late and ended quickly, as in the case of the Benevolent Asylum and the Hospital for Sick Children. Whereas the pattern of onset shows a bimodal

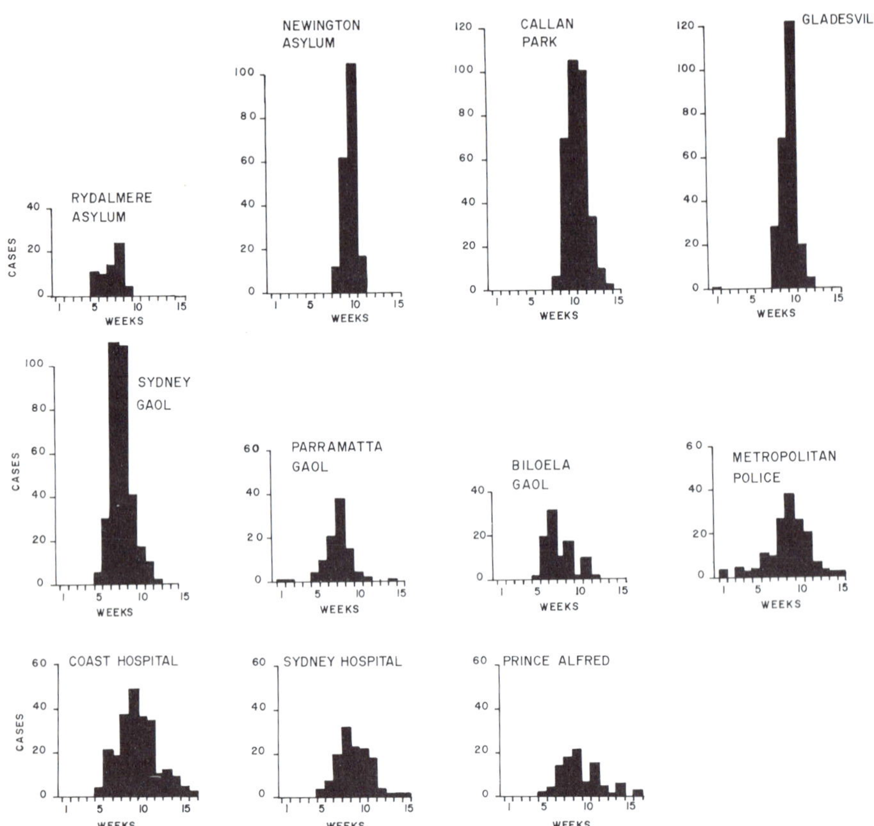

Figure 51 Temporal distribution of influenza cases, Sydney institutions 1891

distribution with peaks in week 5 and weeks 8–9, peak morbidity was largely concentrated in weeks 9–10. The earliest peak occurred amongst the inmates of the Sydney and Biloela Gaols (week 7) followed in week 8 by Rydalmere Hospital, Parramatta Gaol and the Sydney Hospital. The latest peak (week 10) occurred at the Newington, Callan Park and Gladesville Asylums (Table 31).

THE EPIDEMIOLOGICAL IMPACT

In total there were 234 deaths from influenza in Sydney during the 1891 epidemic. At the same time there were approximately 2500 cases of the disease among the inmates and employees of Sydney's main public institutions. In his official report on the 1891 epidemic Ashburton-Thompson estimated that there were in total between 120 000 and 130 000 cases of influenza in New South Wales during the epidemic (Ashburton-Thompson, 1892:7). This figure was arrived at on the basis of the 32 500 cases actually seen by the 148 medical practitioners who replied to his official questionnaire. Ashburton-Thompson simply divided the 32 500 by 148

Table 31 Influenza Experience, Leading Sydney Institutions 1891

Institution	*First case (week)*[a]	*Last case (week)*[a]	*Peak morbidity (week)*[a]
Rydalmere Hospital for Insane	5	9	8
Gladesville Hospital for Insane	5	12	10
Callan Park Hospital for Insane	8	14	10
Newington Asylum	8	11	10
Sydney Gaol	5	12	7
Parramatta Gaol	1	14	8
Biloela Gaol	5	12	7
Coast Hospital	5	16	9
Sydney Hospital	4	15	8
Prince Alfred Hospital	5	16	9
Moorcliffe Hospital	8	12	10
St Vincent's Hospital	6	16	n.a.
Hospital for Sick Children	8	9	n.a.
Ashfield Infants Home	9	n.a.	n.a.
Benevolent Asylum	9	11	9
Metropolitan Police	1	15	9
All institutions	1	16	10

Source: Ashburton-Thompson, 1892.
n.a. No information available.
[a] Schedule of weeks as follows: week 1 — 2–8 Sept.; 2 — 9–15 Sept.; 3 — 16–22 Sept.; 4 — 23–29 Sept.; 5 — 30 Sept–6 Oct.; 6 — 7–13 Oct.; 7 — 14–20 Oct.; 8 — 21–27 Oct.; 9 — 28 Oct.–3 Nov.; 10 — 4–10 Nov.; 11 — 11–17 Nov.; 12 — 18–24 Nov.; 13 — 25 Nov.–1 Dec.; 14 — 2–8 Dec.; 15 — 9–15 Dec.; 16 — 16–22 Dec.

and multiplied the answer by the total number of medical practitioners in the colony (219.6 × 561 = 123 196). It seems highly likely that the numbers who sought formal medical treatment during the epidemic represented only a small proportion of the total numbers affected. Ashburton-Thompson's rather crude estimates would, therefore, seem to understate substantially the total number of people who had influenza in 1891. While no official figures exist it would seem from the experience of Sydney's institutions that the total number of cases was considerably more. Table 32 suggests that for some of Sydney's closed institutions (e.g. Sydney Gaol, Callan Park Asylum, etc.) the number of cases could be as high as 44–7 per cent of the total institutional population. Figures for the open institutions such as the police force indicate a lower proportion but still of the order of 26 per cent. Finally, there are some data recording the number of post office employees absent sick during 1891 (although no details are provided as to the nature of the illness) and these indicate a figure of 26.5 per cent off sick during the epidemic months. If these populations provide a guide to total morbidity it is reasonable to assume that approximately 25–6 per cent of Sydney's population had influenza during 1891. This would give an approximate total of 100 000 cases in the Sydney area alone. If these figures are anywhere near accurate then the influenza epidemic in terms of the total numbers ill rather than actually dying was the greatest epidemic of the nineteenth century. In parts of Sydney the impact of the epidemic in terms of number of people ill was severe. Up to 4 December, for example, it was estimated that there had been 1000 cases of the disease in Penrith

Table 32 Influenza Cases, Sydney's Major Institutions 1891

Institution	*Total cases*[a]	*Population at risk*[a]	*Rate per 100*[a]
Rydalmere Hospital for the Insane	63	142	44.4
Callan Park Hospital for the Insane	325[b]	814[b]	39.9[b]
Gladesville Hospital for the Insane	240	879	27.3
Parramatta Hospital for the Insane	170	1163	14.6
Newington Asylum	196	498	39.3
Sydney Gaol	318	675	47.1
Parramatta Gaol	98[b]	341[b]	28.7[b]
Biloela Gaol	90	202	44.5
Coast Hospital	235[b]	n.a.	
Sydney Hospital	98[c] (36)	(249)	(14.5)
Prince Alfred Hospital	64[c] (27)	(85)	(31.8)
Moorcliffe Hospital	27	60	45.0
St Vincent's Hospital	53	n.a.	
Hospital for Sick Children	3[c] (5)	(42)	(11.9)
Ashfield Infants Home	8	n.a.	
Benevolent Asylum	19	247	7.7
Metropolitan Police	159	604	26.3
Training ship *Vernon*	1	245	0.4

Source: Ashburton-Thompson, 1892.
n.a. No data available.
[a] Staff and inmates unless otherwise stated.
[c] New admissions only.
( ) Staff and/or inmates only.
[b] Inmates only.

Table 33 Death Rates (per 1000) from Influenza by Age and Sex, Sydney 1891

Age group	*Males*	*Females*	*Total*
0–4	0.65	0.37	0.51
5–9	0.17	0.09	0.13
10–14	0.11	0.05	0.07
15–19	0.24	0.11	0.17
20–24	0.16	0.18	0.17
25–29	0.05	0.15	0.10
30–34	0.27	0.52	0.38
35–39	0.50	0.89	0.67
40–44	0.39	0.22	0.30
45–49	0.86	0.55	0.71
50–54	1.42	1.20	1.32
55–59	1.56	2.21	1.87
60–64	2.12	3.53	2.82
65–69	3.23	5.31	4.28
70–74	8.59	10.53	9.63
75–79	17.12	17.11	17.11
80–84	12.45	40.29	27.24
85–89	32.79	23.26	27.21
90 +	32.26	32.25	32.26
Total	0.57	0.65	0.61

Sources: Registrar-General, Death Records, 1891; Census of N.S.W., 1891.

alone, approximately 40 per cent of the area's total population (*SMH*, 4 December 1891:7). By contrast to the morbidity invoked by the epidemic, mortality rates were very low. The overall case fatality rate was only 0.61 per 1000 although, as Table 33 indicates, death rates increased significantly with age. The epidemic had its greatest impact on those over the age of 50 years and those over 70 years of age suffered the heaviest mortality of all. The rate for men in Sydney was lowest between the ages of 20 and 34 years, age groups that exhibited the highest mortality rate in the 1919 epidemic.

SPATIAL IMPACT AND DIFFUSION OF THE EPIDEMIC

When it comes to considering the spatial impact and diffusion of influenza in Sydney in 1891 the lack of any data on actual cases of the disease makes the task of reconstruction very difficult. The onset, peak morbidity and duration of the epidemic among Sydney's institutional population has already been touched upon but this material offers little insight into the spatial impact of the disease or its spread across the city. The available material on deaths during the epidemic is also somewhat misleading. In the first place, the numbers dying from the disease were very small. In the second, the distribution of deaths may simply replicate the spatial distribution of Sydney's elderly, infirm and/or institutionalized population. Finally, the pattern of deaths is not a good indication of the pattern of cases in so far as mortality tended to be highest amongst the city's very young and very old population. Nevertheless, in the absence of all but the most generalized comments regarding the number of cases of influenza and their distribution in 1891, the spatial pattern of deaths (Figure 52) provides at least one insight into the areal impact of the disease. Randwick and Hunters Hill municipalities experienced the highest death rate during the epidemic, explicable in terms of their institutional population. For the remainder of Sydney, it is significant that the disease had its greatest impact on the more peripheral suburbs such as Granville, Ryde, Castle Hill, Lane Cove, Kogarah and Rockdale. Only in the case of St Peters, Five Dock, Darlington, Woollahra and Macquarie ward were older inner parts of the city severely affected.

When it comes to considering the disease's diffusion through Sydney we are considerably hampered by the lack of any detailed information on the spatial distribution of cases. Figure 52, which illustrates the spatial pattern of date of onset, refers only to epidemic deaths and, for the reasons advanced earlier, deaths may present a misleading picture of the epidemic's true spatial progress. The only other material available with which to reconstruct the disease's progress through Sydney relates to the rather contradictory and unsatisfactory responses to the Board of Health's questionnaire relating to the date the epidemic started. The 53 Sydney respondents varied widely in their identification of a starting date, sometimes by up to two months for any one area. Nevertheless this material, although incomplete, does provide some indication of the epidemic's spatial diffusion. Figure 53 presents a spatial view of these responses, mapping not only the earliest commencement date given but also the latest date. It would appear from these maps that the epidemic first appeared in Manly, Glebe, and possibly Petersham and parts of the City of Sydney, from where it spread to Annandale, Balmain,

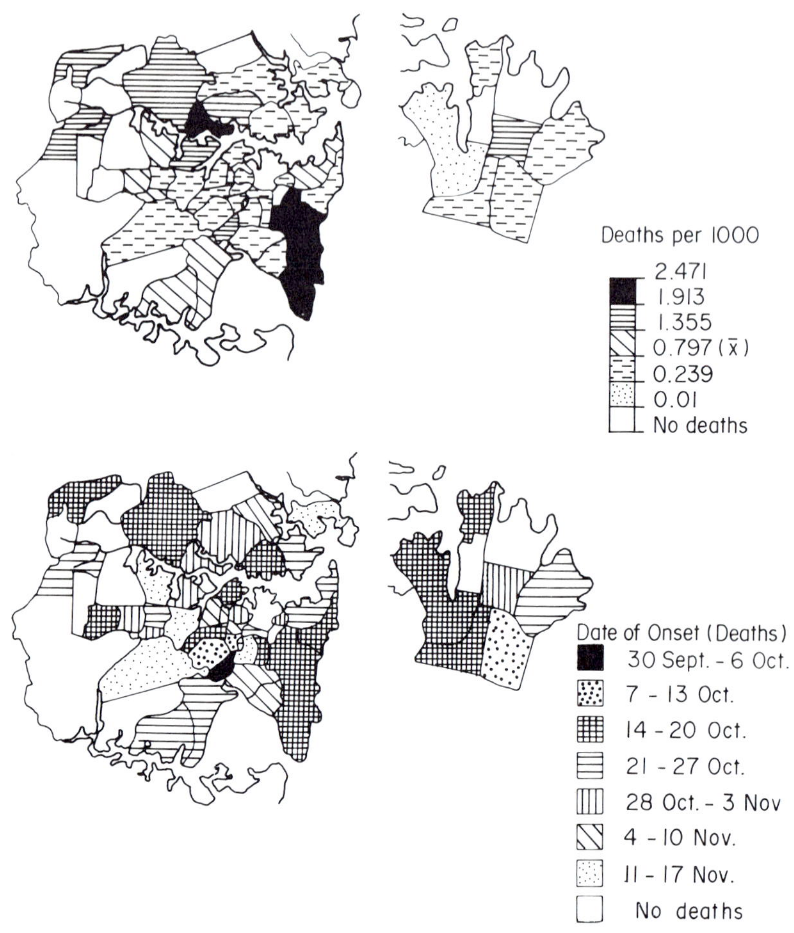

Figure 52 **Influenza deaths per 1000 and date of onset 1891**

North Sydney–Neutral Bay, Woollahra and possibly Waverley and Rockdale. The disease appeared latest in Camperdown, Newtown, Darlington, Erskineville, Paddington and in a series of more suburban municipalities such as Burwood, Hunters Hill, Ashfield and Leichhardt.

DEMOGRAPHIC AND SOCIAL SELECTIVITY

As Figure 54 indicates, the disease was most fatal among persons aged over 50 years by comparison with the 1919 influenza pandemic where the death rate was highest among 25–40-year-olds. In 1891, influenza deaths were predominantly concentrated at the two extremes of life, that is, children under four years and people over 60 years. Together these two groups contributed more than 54 per cent of the total deaths. The number of elderly females to succumb to the disease was also not without significance. Almost 61 per cent of the deaths aged over 60 years and 60 per cent of those aged over 70 years were females. Figure 55 com-

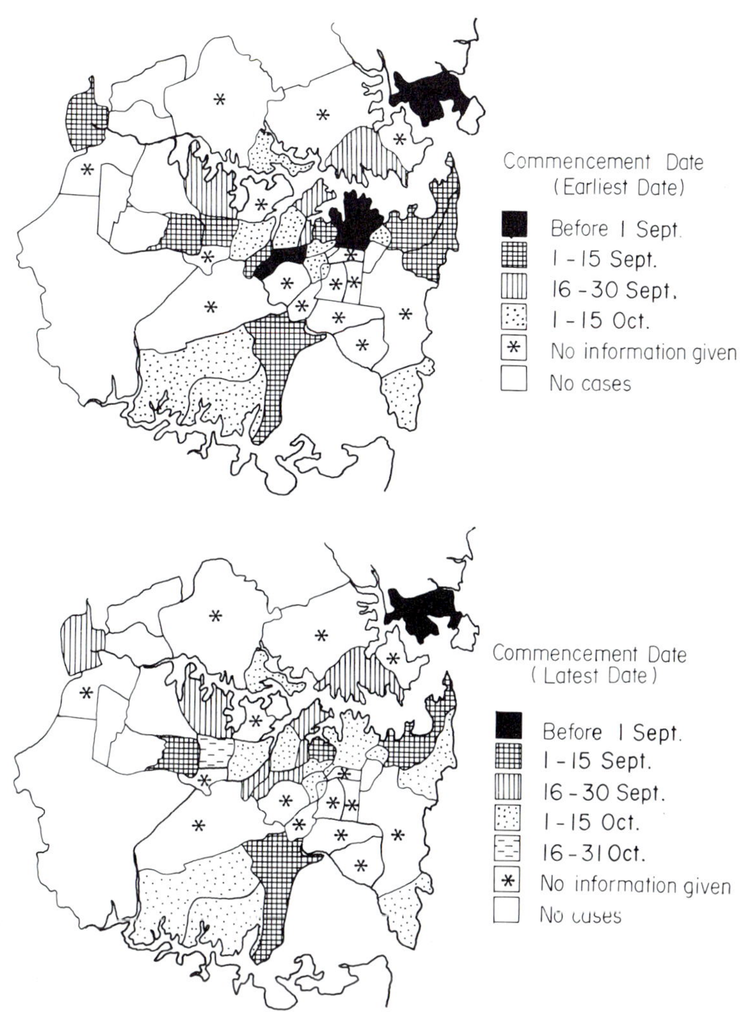

Figure 53 Date of commencement, influenza epidemic 1891

pares the age distribution of deaths during the Sydney epidemic with those that took place in England and Wales during 1891. Basically the two age distributions are almost identical, with proportionally only slightly more deaths under four and over 75 years in Sydney and between 35 and 74 years in England and Wales. The age-sex distribution of deaths provides a somewhat misleading indication of the demographic composition of those who caught the disease. In the first place the elderly and infirm were most at risk of dying from influenza, and in the second, in 1891 females numerically dominated Sydney's elderly population. It would seem, therefore, that the disease was much more widespread through the Sydney community than the age structure of deaths would lead us to believe. Many of the medical respondents to the questionnaire sent out by Ashburton-Thompson indi-

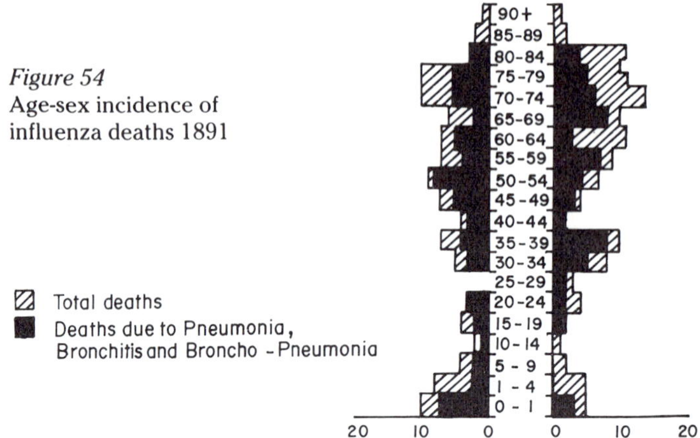

Figure 54
Age-sex incidence of influenza deaths 1891

cated that most of the cases of influenza that they saw were young adults aged between 18 and 40 years.

Table 34 also suggests that apart from the aged and institutional inmates the epidemic affected most of Sydney's social groups fairly equally. Like the measles epidemic of 1867 the infection rate was probably high in all social groups but the aged, infirm and impoverished suffered the highest mortality.

As Table 35 indicates, the major complications leading to death during the epidemic involved secondary bacterial infection of the lower respiratory tract. Sixty-eight per cent of all influenza deaths involved pneumonia, bronchitis or broncho-pneumonia complications, and as Figure 54 shows, the frequency of such complications was greatest in the under one year age group and the age groups between 15 and 60.

OFFICIAL REACTION

When influenza arrived in Sydney in 1890–1 the germ theory of infectious disease was by no means fully accepted by the colony's medical men. Many still held firmly to the belief of miasmas or poisons emanating from dirt and dust and argued that the disease was somehow connected with the inhalation of noxious poisons

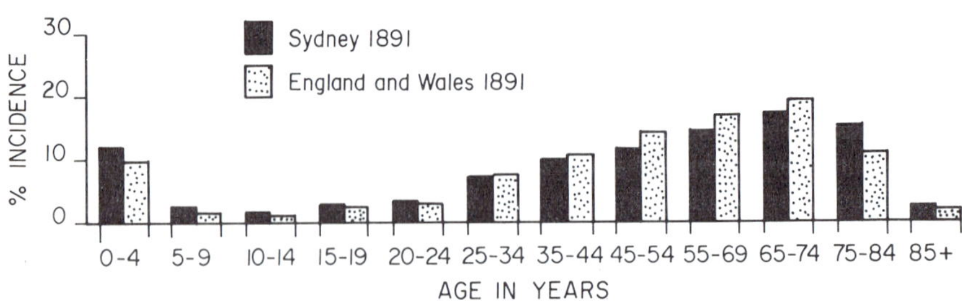

Figure 55 Age-incidence, influenza deaths, Sydney and England and Wales 1891

and was not contagious. One basic problem confronting many of the colony's doctors was that it had been 30 years since the last outbreak of influenza and many were not very familiar with the symptoms, some medical men, to be sure, never having seen a case of the disease. The confusion surrounding influenza is brought home by the responses to the Board of Health's questionnaire where only 178 of the 270 medical respondents were completely convinced that the disease was epidemic influenza rather than a form of seasonal catarrh or some other ailment (Ashburton-Thompson, 1892). Even those doctors who wholeheartedly accepted the germ theory of infectious disease were frustrated by the lack of any firm evidence for a bacterial cause of influenza. Among Ashburton-Thompson and his colleagues the epidemic produced a concentrated effort to establish the causes of the disease and the medium of its spread. The questions that preoccupied Ashburton-Thompson mainly centred on how the disease spread, whether one attack conveyed any degree of immunity, what socio-economic and geographical factors favoured epidemic outbreaks, how long the infective period was, and whether or not there was any medium whereby infection could survive or multiply outside the body. The responses to the Board of Health's questionnaire provide some answers to these questions but were generally contradictory, anecdotal and muddled. What they did demonstrate fairly conclusively, however, was that the disease was spread by person-to-person transmission. When it came to formulating an official policy for handling the epidemic the Board of Health found themselves in something of a quandary. Faced by a disease which in a large number of cases never became easily or certainly identifiable, which was often so mild as to escape detection, which spread rapidly and affected a very large proportion of the total population, the Board found that the methods adopted for the smallpox epidemic such as notification, isolation, quarantine and formal cleansing and fumigation were impossible to put into effect. Consequently official emphasis was placed on a public education campaign and pamphlets and posters were distributed to many householders in the city. Recognizing that the disease was highly communicable

Table 34 Socio-economic Status, Influenza Deaths 1891

Socio-economic group	*Number*	*%*
Unskilled	34	14.5
Semi-skilled	28	12.0
Tradesman	39	16.7
Clerical	14	6.0
Proprietor	18	7.7
Professional/gentleman	7	3.0
Farmer	10	4.2
Scholar	3	1.3
Housewife	15	6.4
Inmate institution	14	6.0
Retired	28	12.0
Other	5	2.1
Not stated (under 65 years)	19	8.1
Total	234	100.0

Source: Registrar-General, Death Records, 1891.

Table 35 Deaths from Complications, Influenza 1891

Major complication	*Number*
Pneumonia	59
Broncho-pneumonia	23
Bronchitis	46
Congestion of lungs	2
Asthma	2
Convulsions	4
Heart disease	3
Diabetes	2
Meningitis	2
Debility	1
Tuberculosis	1
Suicide	1
Other	13
Total	159

Source: Registrar-General, Death Records, 1891.

and spread primarily from the sick to the healthy by airborne droplet the Board decided that the best defence was to encourage people to avoid large gatherings and places of public resort (meetings, public transport, etc.), to refuse to receive visitors when sick and to keep sick children away from school. A circular distributed to many homes in the city urged people to avoid crowds, to avoid speaking at close quarters and 'demonstrative signs of affection', to cover the mouth when coughing, and if it proved necessary to spit, then to do so into a special container carried for the purpose containing disinfectant.

COMMUNITY IMPACT AND PUBLIC REACTION

One measure of the impact of the epidemic was the cost in terms of human misery, the tragedy of sudden bereavement. Although only 234 died as a direct result of influenza it is certain that the disease contributed to many more deaths, particularly heart and chest patients whose deaths were hastened. It was in its extreme morbidity rather than in its mortality, however, that the epidemic caused most disruption to the social and economic life of the metropolis. The fact that so many people caught the disease at the same time played havoc with the city's normal services and activities. Although accurate figures are impossible to obtain it would seem that between 30 and 35 per cent of all government employees, shop assistants and workers caught the disease during October and November. For those who worked in one of the city's many institutions the percentage was even higher. Thus, 24 of the 63 staff at Gladesville Hospital caught the disease as did four of the ten workers at Moorcliffe Hospital and ten of the 26 staff at Biloela Gaol (Table 36). Older senior members of the colony's public service and business world suffered particularly. During late October/early November influenza severely disrupted Sydney's judicial processes and many courts had their sittings postponed or rearranged due to the judge's illness. Many schools were also forced to close or cancel classes because of the absence of many teachers. Ordinary public ser-

Table 36 Influenza Cases, Sydney Institutional Staff 1891

	Total staff	*Number influenza cases*	*% ill*
Sydney Gaol	89	29	32.6
Biloela Gaol	26	10	38.5
Gladesville Hospital	63	24	38.1
Sydney Hospital	63	17	27.0
Prince Alfred Hospital	85	27	31.8
Moorcliffe Hospital	10	4	40.0
Ashfield Hospital for Children	17	5	29.4
Metropolitan Police	604	159	26.3

Source: Ashburton-Thompson, 1892.

vices were hard-pressed to maintain normal activities. On Saturday 31 October, for example, the tramways department had 32 motormen off sick with influenza and rather than cancel any tram services they decided to cease watering Sydney's streets, causing a great outcry about the dusty streets (see *SMH*, 5 November 1891:6).

No aspect of Sydney life escaped the epidemic's heavy hand. People nervously shied away from large gatherings and attendances were greatly reduced at all theatres, church services and sporting events. Only 12 000 turned up on the first day at the Sydney Cricket Ground to see Dr W. G. Grace play in Lord Sheffield's All England team against New South Wales, and when the English team came to play matches against a Parramatta 22 and a Camden 22 rumour had it that the local sides were hard-pressed to put 22 fit and healthy men into the field. On the local scene the epidemic played havoc with the Sydney cricket season and many teams were forced to play short-handed. Not even the Melbourne Cup escaped unscathed. The railways estimated that they were down £1000 in revenue compared with 1890 because of the fall-off in passenger traffic between Sydney and Melbourne for the race carnival. Many concerts and plays had to be postponed because of the illness of the principals. Such happenings caused a general wave of anxiety to spread across the city.

The *Sydney Morning Herald* and the *Daily Telegraph* ran a daily report on the epidemic as well as details of local dignitaries struck down and the disease's progress through the other Australian colonies. People crowded local dispensaries for prescriptions to be made up, such as in the case at Parramatta on 25 October when a vast throng besieged the Parramatta Friendly Societies' Dispensary. It was later rumoured that their medicine was prepared in a wholesale manner in a large tub (see *SMH*, 26 October 1891:5). By early November such was the public's reaction that the Bishop of Sydney drew up a special prayer to be read in all of Sydney's churches. It called upon God to provide speedy relief from the distress stemming 'from the prevalence of widespread and serious illness amongst us' (*SMH*, 7 November 1891:9). In such an environment the advertisers of popular medicines, although somewhat more restrained than they had been during the smallpox outbreak, reaped a bountiful harvest. 'Scottish Oils' were widely canvassed as a sure cure, although only if 'rubbed into the spine and back twice a

Table 37 Influenza Cases, Gladesville Hospital for the Insane 1891

Section of hospital	Population at risk		Influenza cases		Rate per 100		
	Male	*Female*	*Male*	*Female*	*Male*	*Female*	*Total*
Hill Branch							
Patients	209	—	75	—	35.9	—	35.9
Staff	18	—	9	—	50.0	—	50.0
Main building							
Patients	259	275	1	114	0.4	41.4	21.5
Staff	38	34	9	20	23.7	58.8	40.3
Priory							
Patients	39	—	6	—	15.4	—	15.4
Staff	7	—	6	—	85.7	—	85.7
Total							
Patients	507	275	82	114	16.2	41.4	25.1
Staff	63	34	24	20	38.1	58.8	45.4

Source: Ashburton-Thompson, 1892.

day'. Dr Ferrier's Catarrh Snuff and Oertels Tonic Water were also advertised as sure cures, while Washington H. Soul and Co. sold a special unnamed remedy for 2s.6d. and 4s.6d. a bottle which 'effects a sure cure in one or two days'.

INFLUENZA WITHIN AN INSTITUTION – THE GLADESVILLE HOSPITAL FOR THE INSANE IN 1891

During 1891 influenza took a heavy toll of Sydney's institutional population. Most closed institutions such as gaols and mental hospitals, characterized by overcrowding, poor ventilation, inadequate heating and often insanitary living conditions, provided a fertile environment for the rapid dissemination of a highly infectious disease like influenza. In just three weeks from the end of October there were more than 1200 cases of influenza in Sydney's leading institutions. The experience of the Gladesville Hospital for the Insane provides an example of just how devastating an institutional epidemic could be.

Gladesville Hospital consisted of three sections at the time of the influenza epidemic: a main building housing 259 male and 275 female patients and 72 staff, a Hill Branch approximately one-quarter of a mile away with 209 male inmates and 18 attendants, and a small priory also about one-quarter of a mile away providing accommodation for 39 male patients and six staff. Despite their physical separation these three divisions regularly came together for recreational purposes and for Sunday church services, although in both cases male and female patients were not permitted to mingle. There was also a central laundry, run by a number of female patients from the main building.

Although it is not completely clear it would appear that the disease was introduced to the hospital by a number of nurses/attendants who lived outside the institution and commuted to work every day. The first case, a married male attendant in the main building, occurred as early as 6 October but it was not until three weeks later that the epidemic struck with full force. Between 24 October and 18 November 240 cases of influenza occurred, 44 among the staff and almost 200

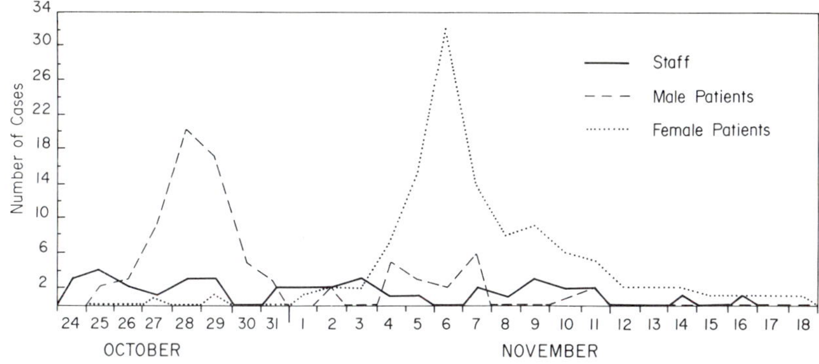

Figure 56 Temporal distribution of influenza cases, Gladesville Asylum 1891

among the inmates. During this time there were six deaths, all but one being elderly females.

As Figure 56 indicates the epidemic came in two waves. Prior to the first wave there appears to have been a mini-outbreak among the hospital staff, particularly those working at the Hill Branch. The epidemic then hit the inmates of this section and between 25 and 31 October 59 male patients caught the disease. A week later the epidemic moved on to affect the main building of the hospital and in the space of seven days more than fifteen cases occurred among the patients and staff. As Figure 56 suggests, the staff may have provided the bridging link between the two distinctive epidemics, although many of the females who worked in the laundry were amongst the first to catch the disease. The laundry served all sections of the hospital and it was usual for soiled linen to be left to accumulate for several days before being washed. Most of the laundry women who caught the disease fell ill during the first few days of November, after which the majority of female patients began to suffer. One of the most intriguing aspects of the epidemic was that the second wave almost exclusively attacked the female wards of the main building, leaving the male wards almost completely unscathed. As Table 37 shows, there was only one case of influenza among the 259 male patients compared to 114 out of 275 female patients. This is even more surprising given the fact that nine of the 38 male attendants in the building went down with the disease.

The answer perhaps lies in the fact that the male wards were located on the opposite side of the building to those of the females and that there was very little internal intermingling or mixing between male and female patients, male attendants and female patients, female nurses and male patients or between attendants and nurses at least during duty hours. Isolation and physical proximity would seem to have been important factors in the spread of the disease. Consequently the 259 male inmates occupied an oasis of immunity while all about them the epidemic raged. In four weeks 240 inmates and staff caught the disease and six patients died. The peak of the epidemic occurred in the week commencing 4 November when 123 cases were notified (see Figure 56). Hardest hit were the female patients and staff in the main building. The morbidity rate among the former was 41.4 per 100, among the latter 58.8. Only the male staff at the Hill

Branch and at the small isolated priory approached these mortality levels. The male staff at the priory were the worst hit of all, six of the seven catching the disease. In addition, most of the family of the attendant-in-charge who lived in the same building caught the disease. Overall, one-quarter of all the inmates of the hospital and 45 per cent of the staff caught influenza during the epidemic. No efforts were made to disinfect the wards involved or to isolate the sufferers until 8 or 9 November, by which time the full force of the epidemic had passed.

CONCLUSIONS

The 1891 influenza pandemic marked the beginning of a new epidemiological era for Sydney. It was the first epidemic to have a general impact on the city's population and although deaths were relatively few it was a morbidity crisis of major proportions. Few Sydney families escaped its effects and the epidemic made a vivid impression on all those who lived through it. The epidemic also caused considerable dislocation to the city's economic and social life and in many places businesses and shops had to close because of lack of staff. Schools and public entertainments in many instances were also forced to close and public gatherings were scrupulously avoided. The epidemic also caused a considerable sense of bewilderment and helplessness in the face of disease on the grand scale.

CHAPTER EIGHT

Pestilence and Poverty

The Plague Epidemic of 1900

BUBONIC PLAGUE is without doubt one of the most fearsome diseases that have afflicted humanity from time to time. Over the last thousand years it has periodically swept out of its traditional homelands in Africa and central Asia to engulf much of the civilized world and has extracted a toll of human life unequalled by that of any other epidemic disease. The epidemic of plague that broke out in Sydney during the late summer of 1900 and ended some seven months later was part of the last great pandemic of plague, which came out of southern China towards the end of last century and which by 1900 had reached most parts of the world. When compared to the celebrated historic outbreaks of plague in the Middle Ages and seventeenth century this pandemic did relatively little to alter the course of human history. Largely it was contained by programmes of quarantine, immunization and improvements in public health. The pandemic did, however, cause great human tragedy and suffering, particularly in Asia where it caused at least ten million deaths. One of the most important effects of this pandemic was that it highlighted shortcomings in urban public health and living conditions in many parts of the world and led to an official inquiry which finally established the aetiology of bubonic plague.

The 1900 epidemic in Sydney was the first major outbreak of this dreaded disease in Australia. It was not to be the last. Between 1900 and 1922 Sydney alone was to experience ten outbreaks of plague with more than 600 cases and 196 deaths (Cumpston and McCallum, 1926). In the context of the developed world there seems little doubt that Australia suffered more than most countries from plague. In the 22 years after 1900 more than 1360 Australians had the misfortune to catch the disease and for 535 it proved fatal. The 1900 epidemic in Sydney had all the ingredients of a major social tragedy. It produced scenes of mass hysteria and panic which surpassed those of the smallpox outbreak 20 years before. It caused a degree of suffering out of all proportion to the numbers actually involved and it caused substantial disruption to the colony's social and economic life. Large areas of central Sydney were closed off to traffic and pedestrians and organized health teams conducted a house-to-house cleansing and fumigation operation. Many businesses were closed and their owners pushed to the edge of financial ruin. Almost 2000 people were forcibly removed from their homes and quarantined at the North Head Quarantine Station. Many private homes and outbuildings were demolished and official teams of rat catchers plied their trade with amazing vigour and resourcefulness. In the face of medical science's inability to cope with the outbreak, people resorted to popular medicines and cures as well as to more traditional measures. People were urged to burn barrels of tar in the streets to purify the air and remove all harmful miasmas. Like the earlier smallpox epidemic neighbour spied upon neighbour and the Chinese were subjected to a virulent campaign of personal abuse and vilification. The columns of the popular press were full of gruesome tales of earlier epidemics as well as day-to-day accounts of plague cases and victims, premises quarantined, people removed, etc. People were reported fleeing their homes, the other Australian colonies boycotted New South Wales goods and quarantined her ships and travellers. Above all the epidemic demonstrated at both a public and private level the intense reaction of people confronted by a disease with the historical connotations of bubonic plague. It also, like the smallpox epidemic of 1881–2, exemplified the irrationality and stubbornness of human behaviour and the almost commanding need to seek refuge in traditional explanations and solutions.

THE EPIDEMIOLOGY OF PLAGUE

Plague is a disease surrounded by myth and half-truths. It is only relatively recently that the actual mechanisms of its transmission and aetiology have been fully understood. The plague bacillus was first isolated by Yersin in 1894 and the detailed epidemiology of the disease established by Hankin, Simond and Ogata in the period 1897–1900 (see Hirst, 1953). Despite this and subsequent work many ambiguities remain. Even today it is not unusual for cases to escape detection or defy diagnosis, as a number of other diseases mimic human plague symptoms.[1]

The epidemiology of plague is extremely complex. There are a multiplicity of factors involved which influence the balance that exists between the preservation of natural reservoirs of the disease and the degree of risk to which human beings are exposed. The progress of any epidemic is strongly affected by a variety of ecological and socio-economic factors governing the life-style and activity pattern of fleas, rodents and humans. Crucial in the maintenance of an urban epidemic would seem to be such factors as high population densities, depressed living conditions, poor sanitation and the juxtaposition of wharf/warehouse and residential areas. In their turn, both flea and rodent are affected by a variety of physical and environmental factors. Bubonic plague is a flea-borne bacterial disease that occurs in nature as an interstitial parasite of small ground-living animals. Primarily, plague is a disease of wild animals, a zoonosis, which is only infrequently

[1] Diseases such as cat scratch fever, tularema, anthrax, mumps and diphtheria can produce symptoms in humans very much akin to bubonic plague.

transmitted to humans. It would appear to be just one of a series of natural diseases well adapted to the seasonal rhythm of such animals that from time to time reaches epidemic proportions (an epizootic) and it is during such epizootics that human beings and their domestic animals are placed at most risk of infection (Pollitzer, 1954:500). Humans are thus infected accidentally via the medium of infected fleas living on domestic or commensal rats. Fleas, therefore, act as the medium of transmission of the disease both from rodents to rodents and from rodents to humans. The frequency of transmission is governed by a wide variety of factors determining the life-style and ecology of fleas, rodents and humans. The element of chance, however, plays a major role in the transmission-infection cycle.

Despite its dreaded reputation and wide geographical distribution, bubonic plague is not a common disease among human communities. Three particular forms of plague are known to exist. Bubonic plague is the most common variety and derives its name from the swollen and inflammed lymph glands (buboes) commonly in the groin, armpit or neck. If not treated, the bacteria invade the circulatory system and associated organs, and death may result from heart failure in about five to seven days. The mortality rate from bubonic plague varies widely but during severe epidemics can reach 40 to 90 per cent. The second form of plague takes the character of a septicaemic infection. During a particularly virulent outbreak of the disease, plague bacteria proliferate so quickly as to overwhelm the body's defences and cause death within 24 hours. Occasionally, the plague bacteria involve the lungs by inciting or exploiting secondary pneumonia and producing what is termed 'pneumonic plague'. This remains the most dreaded and contagious of all plague forms. Independently of rodents it spreads directly from person to person by air-borne droplets produced during coughing, sneezing or speaking. While the detailed epidemiology of this form of plague is still uncertain it remains one of the deadliest diseases known, with a case fatality rate of near 100 per cent unless treated within hours of onset. Fortunately, this particular variant occurs only rarely. The most important outbreak of pneumonic plague in recent times occurred in Manchuria and northern China in 1910–11 and produced more than 60 000 deaths. Australia has remained free of pneumonic plague although there appear to have been several cases in Maryborough, Queensland in 1905 (Ham, 1907:56–9).

The residents of Sydney in 1900 had no idea of the different types of plague nor did they understand the epidemiology of the disease or the manner of its transmission. In so far as they thought about such things they probably believed that the disease was spread by direct contact with an infected person, probably a Chinese person. As to Sydney's medical men, opinion was divided. Some accepted the recently formulated rat-flea theory of dissemination while others, while accepting a bacterial origin, argued that the disease was primarily gastro-intestinal and spread by personal contact. A few still clung to the older belief that the disease arose from filth, impure air and insanitary living conditions. The rat-flea explanation of the disease's transmission was very new in 1900, having been advanced only a year or two before by Hankin and Simond. Hankin concluded that the incidence of plague stood in close relation to the accessibility of rats to human households and that some intermediary insect was necessary to communicate the disease from rat to human. Simond, working in India, formulated the flea hypothesis to account for this intercommunication of plague between rat and human. During the Sydney epidemic the connection between plague in rats and plague in humans was accepted almost from the outset by Ashburton-Thompson, the chief medical officer of health. Ashburton-Thompson, whose official report on the epidemic remains one of the classic epidemiological reports of the last hundred years, almost at once embraced the rat-flea theory, and his report provides much circumstantial evidence to support the view of the disease being spread by fleas (see Ashburton-Thompson, 1901). He also appreciated the fact that an epizootic of plague among rats invariably preceded an epidemic in humans. On epidemiological grounds alone he seems to have regarded the existence of an intermediary between the rat and human beings as essential. Frank Tidswell, the official New South Wales government bacteriologist, was one of the first people to recognize that a special rat-flea was implicated in spreading the disease, even though he initially made the mistake of thinking that it was the dog and cat flea that was responsible (Ashburton-Thompson, 1903:71). Ashburton-Thompson's work on the epidemic established among other things that there existed a close association between plague in rats and plague in humans, that an epizootic always preceded an epidemic, and that the incidence of rats and human plague was heaviest during the months of April, May and June. Recognition of such things was one matter; however, convincing the government, local authorities and the general public was something else entirely.

Unfortunately we may never know precisely from where the 1900 epidemic arrived in Sydney. In the years immediately preceding the outbreak plague was epidemic in at least half a dozen port cities all in regular contact with Sydney. The disease could have been introduced to Australia from any one of a number of cities such as Bombay, Hong Kong, Calcutta, Singapore, Mauritius, Honolulu or Noumea. Between late October 1899 and January 1900 at least thirteen ships from plague-infested ports were berthed at the Darling Harbour or Central wharves in Sydney (Ashburton-Thompson, 1901:22). Suffice it to say that the first case of plague was a carman whose job regularly involved him in handling parcels from the above wharves. He fell ill on 19 January. The subsequent epidemic gripped the city from late February until mid-August. During this period 303 people caught plague, 103 never to recover. The peak of the epidemic was reached during a five-week period in late April/early May (Figure 57) during which time 40 per cent of all cases (120) and 50 per cent of all deaths occurred. Overall, the epidemic was at its most severe from late March until the second week of May (weeks 10–17 on Figure 57) and this period produced 69 per cent of all cases and 61 per cent of all deaths. By early May it appeared as if the epidemic was waning but in an ironic twist of fate a reprise occurred in mid-May and lasted until the end of June (weeks 18–23). By the end of June it was at last clear that the outbreak was almost over despite a handful of isolated cases and deaths that extended until mid-August.

ONSET AND PEAK

Figure 58 shows the spatial sequence of onset by place of work and place of residence. For place of work plague appeared earliest in The Rocks (Gipps ward) followed by the wards immediately to the south (Brisbane and Denison), Redfern

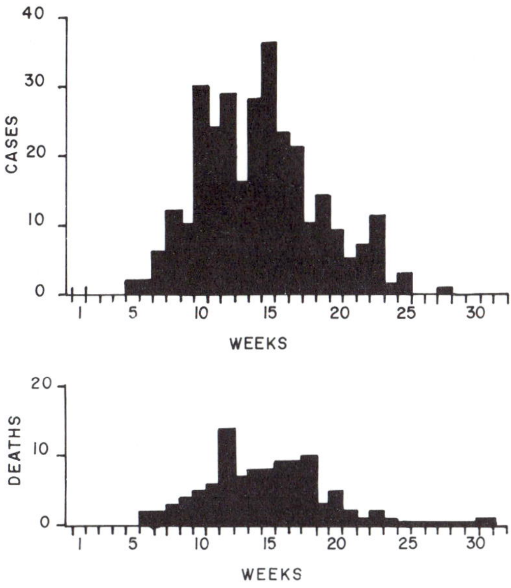

Figure 57 Temporal distribution of plague cases and deaths 1900

and Glebe. By the end of March, plague had also appeared in Bourke and Macquarie and Phillip wards, Annandale and Leichhardt. The second week of April saw a considerable expansion of the disease with plague penetrating a group of suburbs in the inner west and southwest as well as Fitzroy ward and Woollahra to the east. The areas of the metropolis where plague appeared latest were generally on the North Shore and in the south. By place of residence the pattern of onset differs somewhat from that of place of work. The earliest appearance of the disease was in The Rocks, Denison ward, Redfern, Glebe and Annandale, the latest in Alexandria, Hurstville, Burwood, Marsfield and Wahroonga.

The peak period of morbidity (based on highest fortnightly case totals by place of work) shows that generally the period of highest incidence occurred earliest for people working in Redfern, Brisbane ward, Leichhardt and Darlington. In some areas, although the disease appeared early it peaked late, such as in The Rocks (Gipps ward) and much of the remainder of the City of Sydney (Figure 59).

DURATION OF THE EPIDEMIC

In time as well as space the epidemic had a differential effect on Sydney. Although plague was present in the City for 29 weeks not all parts of the metropolitan area experienced such a long visitation. As Figure 58 illustrates, plague lingered longest in parts of the central city, notably Glebe, The Rocks (Gipps ward), Annandale, Denison and Cook wards, Redfern, Paddington and Balmain. The disease's shortest visitation was in the peripheral suburbs such as Randwick, Guildford,

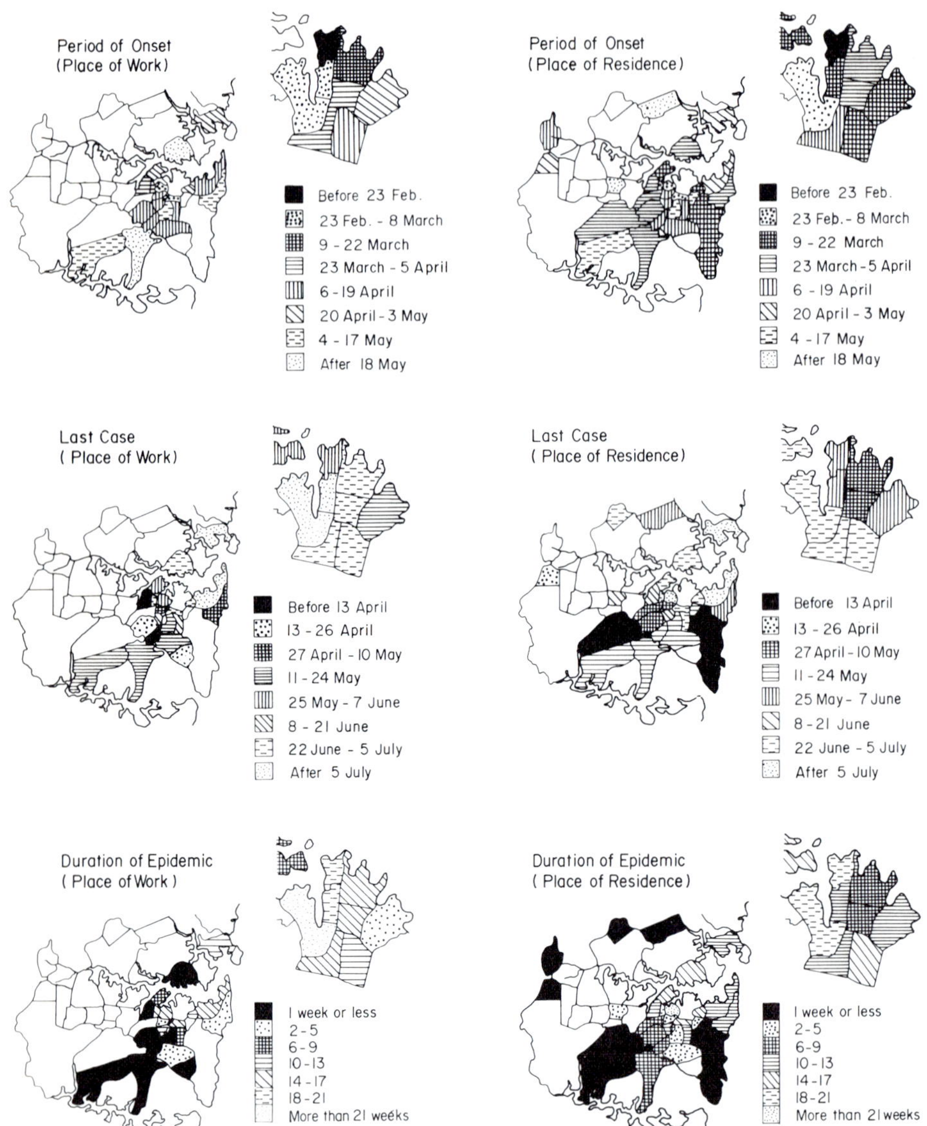

Figure 58 Period of onset, last case and duration of epidemic, plague 1900

Canterbury and Marsfield as well as in some inner-city areas as Camperdown, Alexandria and North Botany. For such areas plague was a temporary inconvenience, albeit a most unwelcome and unpleasant one.

SPATIAL DISTRIBUTION

The plague epidemic was also concentrated geographically and here it is valuable to distinguish between the victim's place of residence and place of work. Gener-

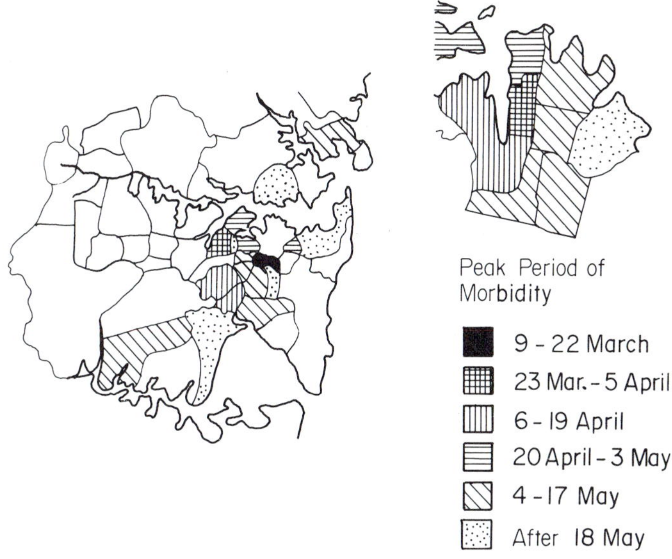

Figure 59 **Peak period of morbidity, plague epidemic 1900**

ally, the epidemic hit the wharf and central business areas of Sydney hardest and those employed therein and/or living nearby suffered greatly. Where a person worked in 1900 Sydney probably in the long run had more to do with whether he or she caught plague than did place of residence. When place of work is considered, the City of Sydney and especially the area located between Darling Harbour, George Street and Central Railway Station vividly stands out as the major focus of the epidemic (Figure 60). More than 60 per cent of all cases worked somewhere within this broad area. By place of residence the worst affected areas of the metropolis lay in that part of central Sydney bounded by the Darling Harbour wharves, Elizabeth Street and the Haymarket as well as parts of Surry Hills, Redfern, Waterloo, Paddington, Camperdown, Glebe and Balmain. Together these areas accounted for 70 per cent of all cases and deaths. In terms of place of residence the disease was at its most virulent in the streets of Lang ward, the closely packed, depressed residential tenements fronting Darling Harbour.

The explanation of such a spatial concentration of plague lies in the social geography of Sydney. The area worst affected formed the nucleus of Sydney's social and economic life. Here were to be found most of the city's produce and provision merchants, warehouses, shops and business houses as well as many small factories, foundries, mills, hotels and offices. In addition, Darling Harbour was a major focus not only of overseas and coastal shipping services but also of the city's suburban passenger network. Residentially this area provided accommodation for Sydney's more cosmopolitan and disadvantaged residents, more often than not in undistinguished, depressed housing. Wharf labourers, seamen, unskilled workers, shopkeepers and self-employed tradesmen lived cheek-by-jowl in tiny timeworn cottages or crowded tenements and boarding houses. There is

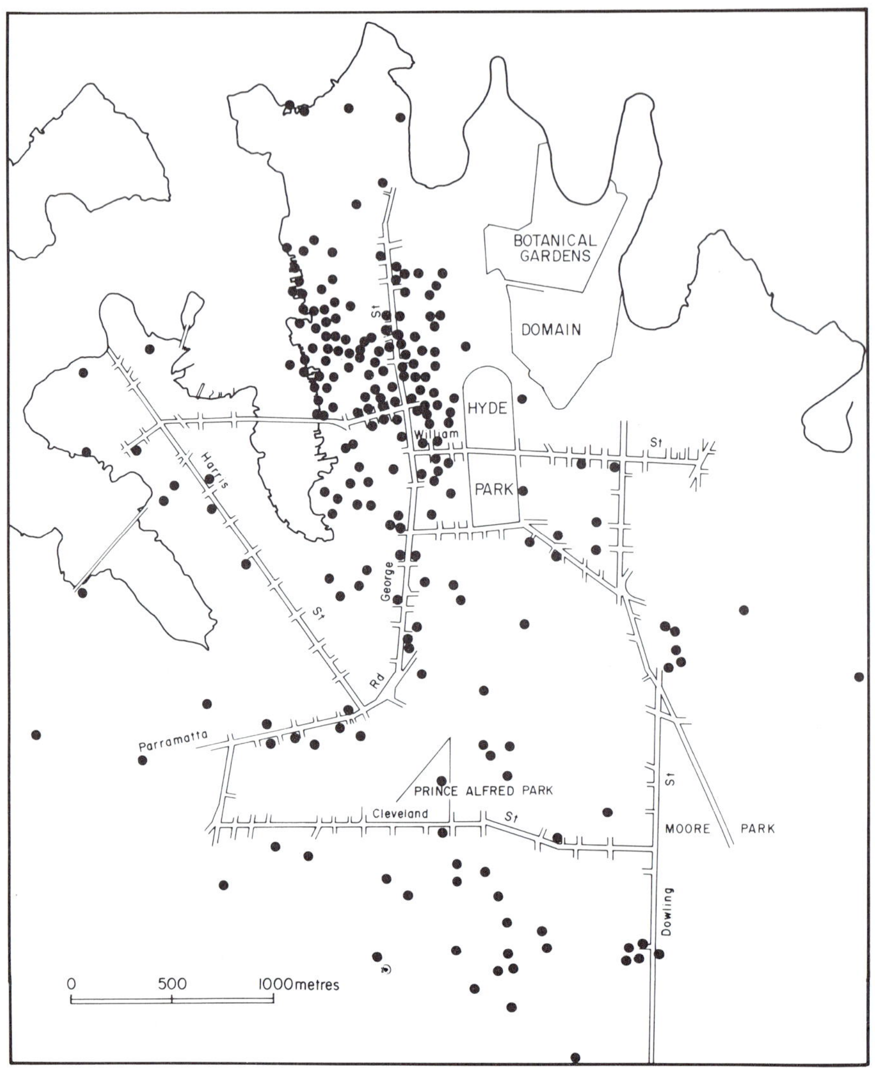

Figure 60 Distribution of plague cases, City of Sydney 1900

little doubt that living and working conditions were overcrowded, unhygienic and insanitary and that even at the best of times the area supported a large rat population. The social geography of Sydney clearly indicates that plague, poverty and centrality were closely associated. There were several reasons for this. In the first place, the disease was highly selective in terms of those it affected. Most of those who caught plague were working-class males plus a handful of self-employed who lived and worked in central Sydney. The middle and upper classes were almost completely untouched by the epidemic. At one level the disease fell heaviest on those males working at or in close association with the central city produce trade

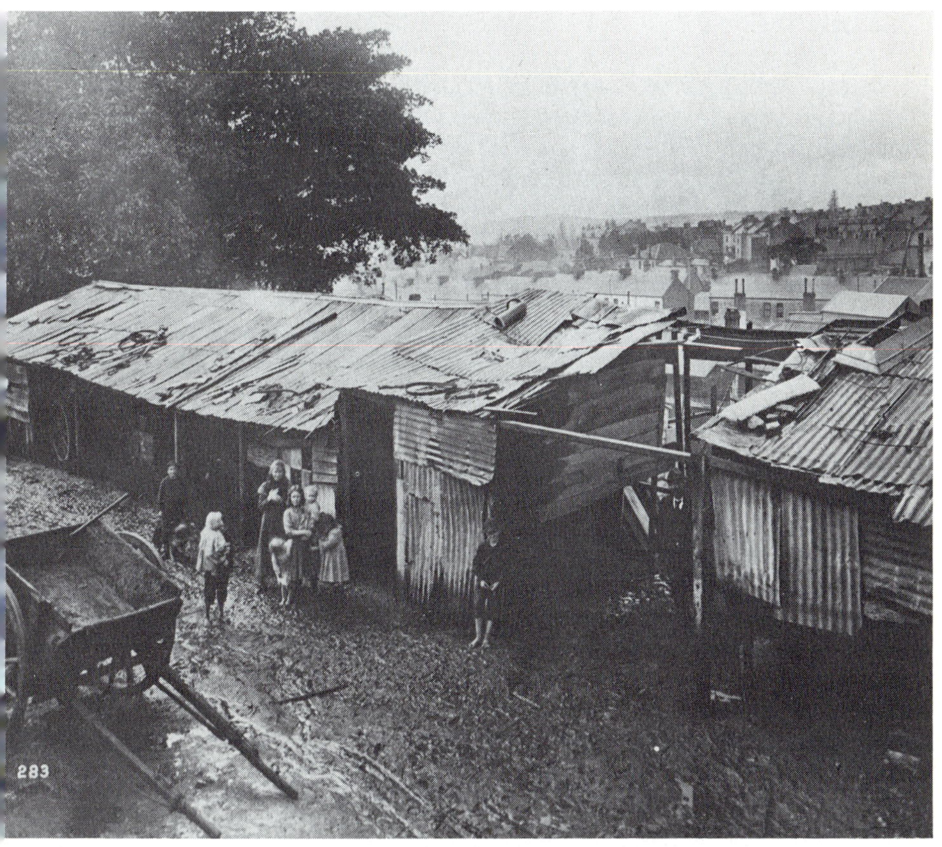

Stables at the rear of 30–2 Oxford Street, Paddington. Plague-infected rats were often transported in bags of feed to such establishments, causing small localized outbreaks of plague.
McCreadie File, Mitchell Library, Sydney

in hay, chaff, maize and potatoes as well as with a variety of other goods and materials handled through the Darling Harbour wharves and warehouses. At another level, it affected those who by the nature and location of their work came into regular daily contact with the above — people such as hotel and restaurant workers, butchers, bakers, carters, draymen and the like. Finally, at a third level plague affected those who worked in a variety of suburban factories and stores which were reliant on the central wharves and warehouses for their supplies and raw materials. In some instances the disease was taken home by such workers and subsequently introduced to family and friends.

In the second place, plague was also a consequence of the severely depressed and insanitary living and working conditions of Sydney's poor. Their housing was dilapidated and crowded together, their homes harboured more rats and their clothes and personal effects more fleas. In a large number of cases their housing was located close to central wharves and warehouses — the major focus of the epidemic. The residential streets bordering Darling Harbour were undoubtedly the worst off in these respects. Many houses were structurally in need of repair and suffered from a lack of adequate ventilation, perpetual dampness and a great accumulation of filth and rubbish. The majority lacked even the most basic sanitary and washing facilities. Communal or shared facilities were common, with waste products often ending up in the harbour by way of the street and open drains. Bald statistics fail to convey adequately the wretchedness of living conditions in this central area. For the majority of inhabitants everyday conditions were hazardous, placing individuals and their families consistently at the risk of infection and death. Such circumstances were not confined to the innermost residential areas of the city. Parts of Redfern, Surry Hills, Waterloo and Botany were as bad if not worse. If nothing else, the plague epidemic drew close attention to the shortcomings of Sydney's housing and sanitary situation, particularly as it existed in the inner-city area. It also highlighted the apparent inability of the central and local authorities to do anything to improve the situation. In 1900 there were no uniform building regulations applying to the whole of Sydney, with the result that it was possible to erect and maintain a dwelling without heed to normal sanitation or water. In addition, most of the homes in the City of Sydney remained unsewered and were dependent upon a network of cesspits which honeycombed the inner city.

THE SPATIAL PROGRESS OF THE EPIDEMIC

The progress of the epidemic in time has already been discussed. Its progress in space may be appreciated from Figures 61 and 62 which present a broad fortnightly picture of the plague's movement across the various parts of Sydney.[2] In the weeks following the end of February, plague diffused from its original harbourside focus in a linear and radial fashion following Sydney's major arterial routeways, in some cases to establish mini-foci in suburbs such as Manly, Redfern, Waterloo and Glebe. In broad terms plague spread in a wave-like motion away from the Darling Harbour wharves to engulf surrounding residential areas. This movement was given some direction by the passive transport of rats and fleas in consignments of produce, goods and rubbish from the central warehouses and wharves. It was also undoubtedly helped by the intensive fumigation and cleansing operation around the Darling Harbour wharves which must have driven the rat population further inland in search of refuge. The daily journey to and from work as well as a variety of social and recreational journeys added another dimension. Many people were infected by virtue of their place of work, others from an incidental encounter in the course of their routine daily activities. Plague progressed through the city in a highly irregular and erratic fashion, affecting some areas while completely missing others, in some cases backtracking at a later date. For many, infection depended upon a chance encounter with an infected flea.

By the beginning of May a separate focus had become established at Manly on Sydney's North Shore. Manly was a small village of approximately 3000 people,

[2] This analysis is based on cases of plague by place of residence. For maps of the diffusion of the epidemic based on place of work see Appendix 3.

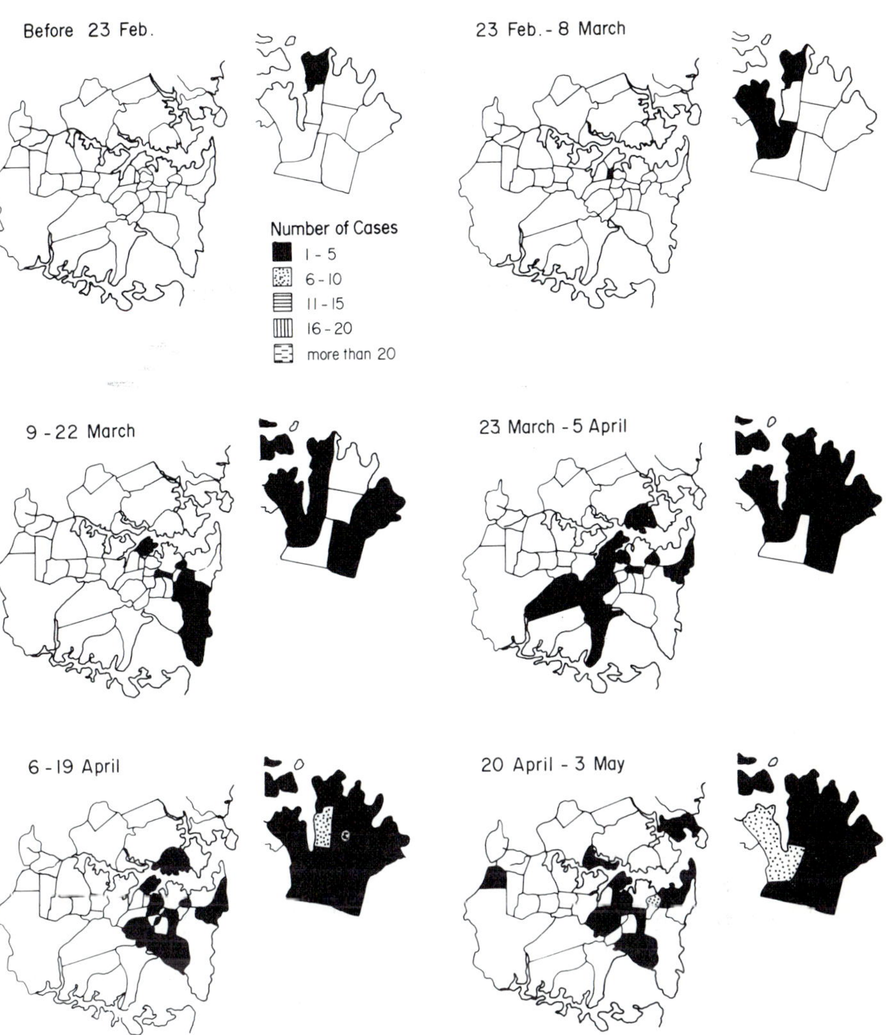

Figure 61 Spatial diffusion of plague cases, February–May 1900

much favoured as a weekend resort by Sydneysiders. The major link with Sydney was by ferry which ran regularly to Darling Harbour. Due to an administrative oversight the ferry avoided being fumigated during the epidemic with the result that infected rats were transported in goods to Manly pier. In the following two months, nine cases of plague appeared, all closely related to the pier site.

In the two weeks after 23 March the epidemic gathered full momentum. All the City of Sydney with the exception of Phillip ward was by now infected and plague had penetrated as far as North Sydney and Waverley. The largest spatial extension,

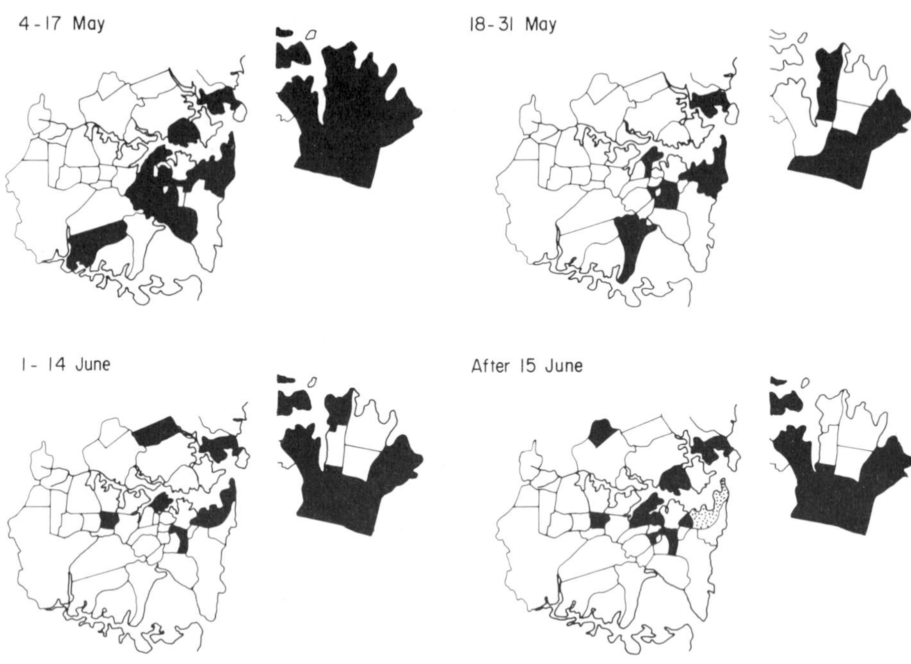

Figure 62 Spatial diffusion of plague cases, May–June 1900

however, had taken place to the west and southwest. By the first week of April plague was present in a continuous belt of suburbs stretching from Balmain, Leichhardt and Annandale through Petersham and Marrickville to Canterbury and Rockdale in the south. In many cases particular suburban outbreaks of the disease could trace their origin to factories or other establishments having received their supplies from downtown wharves and warehouses, for example the Annandale Jam Factory, flour mills and a brewery at Paddington and a rope works at Waterloo. The inference is of course that infected rats and fleas accompanied such supplies on their suburban journeys. Rarely, however, did such outbreaks lead to more than a handful of cases, suggesting that the infection soon died out unless continually resupplied from the city centre. As Figures 61 and 62 show, plague did not diffuse in an orderly way through Sydney but rather in an erratic, discontinuous fashion. Apart from the City of Sydney and a group of inner suburbs such as Glebe, Redfern, Camperdown, Newtown, Paddington and Balmain, plague was present one week, absent the next, only to recur at a later date. By early May the disease had reached its widest areal extent, being present in all parts of the City of Sydney, at Manly and North Sydney on the North Shore, and in a continuous belt of suburbs stretching from Waverley and Woollahra in the east through Paddington, Redfern and Glebe to Balmain, then south to include Petersham, Marrickville, St Peters, Alexandria, Botany and Hurstville. It was a watershed; never again was the disease to achieve such a widespread distribution.

Table 38 Age-Sex Structure, Cases and Deaths, Plague 1900

	Cases			*Deaths*		
Age groups	*Males*	*Females*	*Total*	*Males*	*Females*	*Total*
0–4	5	5	10	4	—	4
5–9	13	7	20	1	3	4
10–14	9	10	19	—	4	4
15–19	52	6	58	18	2	20
20–24	39	7	46	12	1	13
25–29	29	4	33	14	—	14
30–34	17	5	22	3	1	4
35–39	26	4	30	11	—	11
40–44	17	5	22	3	1	4
45–49	13	3	16	7	1	8
50–54	8	—	8	4	—	4
55–59	5	2	7	5	1	6
60–64	2	3	5	1	2	3
65–69	2	3	5	1	2	3
70–74	2	—	2	1	—	1
Total	239	64	303	85	18	103

Source: Register of Cases of Bubonic Plague, 1900.

SOCIAL AND DEMOGRAPHIC SELECTIVITY

Plague attacked nearly four times as many males as females in 1900 and killed nearly five times as many. The reasons for this situation lay in the nature of Sydney's demographic and socio-economic structure and in the location of the outbreak. As mentioned earlier the disease fell mainly on the wharf and adjacent areas and consequently those employed and/or living in these areas suffered the heaviest morbidity and mortality. Males comprised a disproportionate share of Sydney's central workforce in 1900 as well as a substantial proportion of the central residential population. Thus it was largely because males were more at risk due to the location and nature of their job together with their place of residence that explains their higher mortality. Most of those who caught plague were aged between 15 and 45 years (Table 38). The epidemic particularly affected teenage and young adult males. Almost 60 per cent of all cases and deaths were young men aged between 15 and 45 years. Almost 50 children under the age of 15 years were also affected, with 12 deaths. Most of these cases occurred among families living close to the Darling Harbour wharves.

Plague was also highly selective in terms of those occupational groups it affected. Most at risk were males who worked or lived near the Darling Harbour wharves or adjacent streets. Consequently wharf labourers, workers in central provision and produce stores, printing workers, warehousemen and a variety of workers providing retail and recreational services for the central workforce suffered the heaviest morbidity and mortality (Table 39). Outside the central area those who suffered most were the employees of timber merchants, flour mills, breweries, stables and fruiterers that received their raw materials and supplies from the central city wharves and warehouses.

Table 39 Cases and Deaths by Occupational Group, Plague 1900

Occupation	*Cases*	*Deaths*
Produce/provision merchants	32	11
Restaurant/hotel workers	24	9
Tradesmen	25	13
Printers/printing workers	29	7
Wharf labourers/seamen	15	6
Other labourers	19	6
Warehouse workers	18	1
Shop assistants/clerical	12	4
Flour mill/brewery/ wool store/foundry workers	11	1
Housewives	21	9
Children	43	11
Carters/carriers	7	3
Timber merchants	6	4
Unemployed	15	5
Other	31	8
Not stated	5	5
Total	303	103

Source: Register of Cases of Bubonic Plague, 1900.

THE DEMOGRAPHIC IMPACT

Possibly some cases of plague were hidden away or misdiagnosed but the fact remains that in terms of cases and deaths the epidemic had only a very slight impact upon Sydney's demographic structure. Rather its main impact was at a psychological level, particularly in terms of the overtones of panic, hysteria and horror that the disease carried with it. This then was as much an epidemic in people's minds as it was in demographic terms. Both incidence and mortality rates were exceedingly low. As Table 40 indicates, the overall mortality rate was only 2.1 per 10 000 and the incidence rate was 6.2 per 10 000. With respect to males the incidence rate was highest between 15 and 29 years, with the 15–19 age group having a rate of 21.8 per 10 000. Females showed a much lower rate at all age groups and only in the 60–69 year age group did their rate approach that of males. In terms of mortality, males had an overall rate five times that of females. The highest mortality for males was found in the 55–59 year age group (8.1) followed by 15–19-year-olds (7.5) and 25–29-year-olds (7.1).

OFFICIAL REACTION

Once Sydney was officially acknowledged to be an infected city central and local authorities moved quickly to try to contain the outbreak. In this they were undoubtedly assisted by the location of the epidemic. Its concentration amidst the central parts of the city and amongst the working-class population allowed the adoption of more draconian measures than might otherwise have been possible. Official policy took three major forms: (1) the isolation and formal quarantine of all plague cases and contacts, (2) the formal cleansing and fumigation of infected

Table 40 Incidence and Mortality Rates, Plague 1900

	Incidence rate[a]			Mortality rate[b]		
Age group	*Males*	*Females*	*Total*	*Males*	*Females*	*Total*
0–4	2.0	2.0	2.0	1.6	—	0.8
5–9	4.7	2.6	3.7	0.4	1.1	0.7
10–14	3.3	3.6	3.4	—	1.4	0.7
15–19	21.8	2.3	11.6	7.5	0.8	4.0
20–24	17.8	2.6	10.5	5.5	0.4	2.7
25–29	14.7	2.7	8.6	7.1	—	3.2
30–34	9.1	2.5	5.7	1.6	0.5	1.0
35–39	13.3	2.2	8.9	5.6	—	2.9
40–44	10.1	3.4	7.0	1.8	0.7	1.3
45–49	10.6	2.9	8.1	5.7	1.0	3.6
50–54	9.2	—	5.7	4.6	—	2.4
55–59	8.1	3.1	6.6	8.1	1.6	4.8
60–64	4.1	6.0	6.1	2.1	4.0	3.1
65–69	5.7	8.1	8.0	2.8	5.4	4.2
70–74	9.8	—	4.8	4.9	—	2.4
Total[c]	9.9	2.6	6.2	3.5	0.7	2.1

Source: Register of Cases of Bubonic Plague, 1900; Census of N.S.W., 1901.
[a] Cases per 10 000 persons.
[b] Deaths per 10 000 persons.
[c] Only persons aged 0–74 years are included in the calculation of the total incidence rate.

houses and buildings, and (3) an extensive rat extermination campaign. In addition, an effort was made to vaccinate all those who were most at risk from the disease and special facilities and hospitals were established to deal with the outbreak. The policy of isolation and quarantine was also extended to all overseas shipping arrivals.

ISOLATION AND QUARANTINE

As well as actual plague cases the government decreed from the outset the strict isolation and quarantine of all people who had in any way come into contact with plague victims. This indiscriminate removal of both cases of the disease and their contacts continued throughout the epidemic despite representations from the Board of Health that only actual cases should be quarantined. Cases and contacts were removed to the Quarantine Station at North Head. During the epidemic more than 1800 people were officially quarantined. The peak of such compulsory transfers came in late April when in the course of two weeks more than 460 people were forcibly removed from their homes. Both plague victims and contacts were expected to vacate their homes at any hour and were transported by wagonette to the Woolloomooloo quarantine depot. From there they were transported to North Head aboard small steam launches. Frequently no attempt was made to segregate cases from contacts on the journey and one can imagine the terror that must have marked the transfer of many unfortunates. In some cases where people were reluctant to leave their homes they had to be forcibly ejected by the police

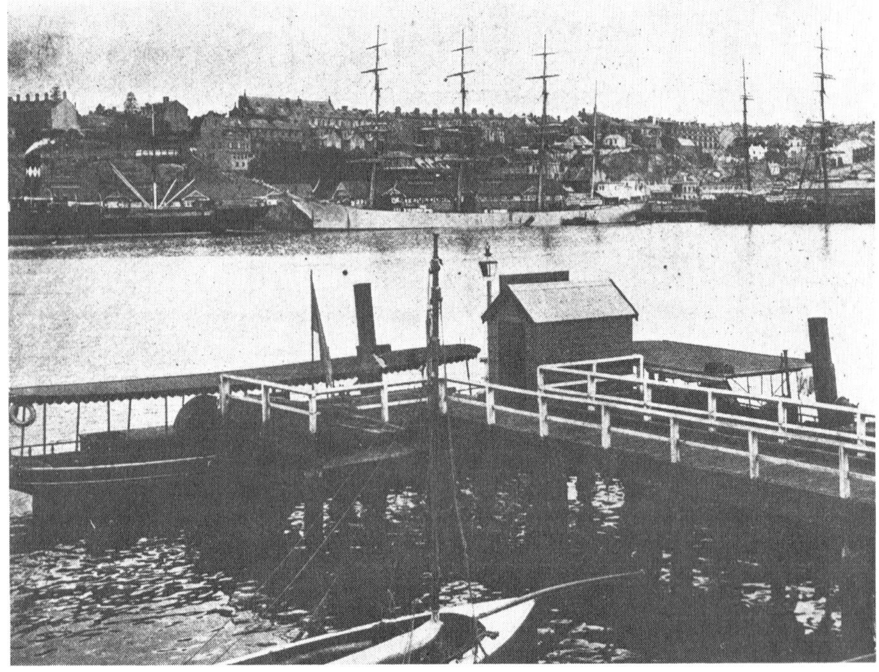

The quarantine wharf, Woolloomooloo Bay.
Town and Country Journal, *31 March 1900. From the original in the General Reference Library, State Library of New South Wales*

and health authorities. In the case of downtown boarding houses and hotels a case or suspected case of plague meant the mass evacuation of dozens of people at a moment's notice. Such was the situation at the Grosvenor Hotel at the end of April when 80 people were forcibly removed following the discovery of a housemaid with plague. Understandably, most people were unwilling to leave their homes for the prospect of an unknown period of detention at North Head. Often there were violent confrontations between the police and health authorities and the luckless cases or contacts.

At the Quarantine Station conditions were a vast improvement on the days of the 1881–2 smallpox epidemic. Food was wholesome and plentiful, living quarters were generally clean and comfortable and medical care and nursing readily available. In addition, each inmate was allowed to send at least one free telegram to Sydney each day. Cases of plague were strictly segregated from contacts. The former were housed in the hospital buildings isolated on the promontory, while contacts were accommodated in detached pavilion-style cottages. The Chinese, viewed with suspicion from the outset, were forced to occupy tents near the beach. Initially it was intended that the period of quarantine should be short, but in practice many were detained for lengthy periods. The average time spent in quarantine for those who actually caught the disease was seven weeks although for some unfortunate people the period was much longer.

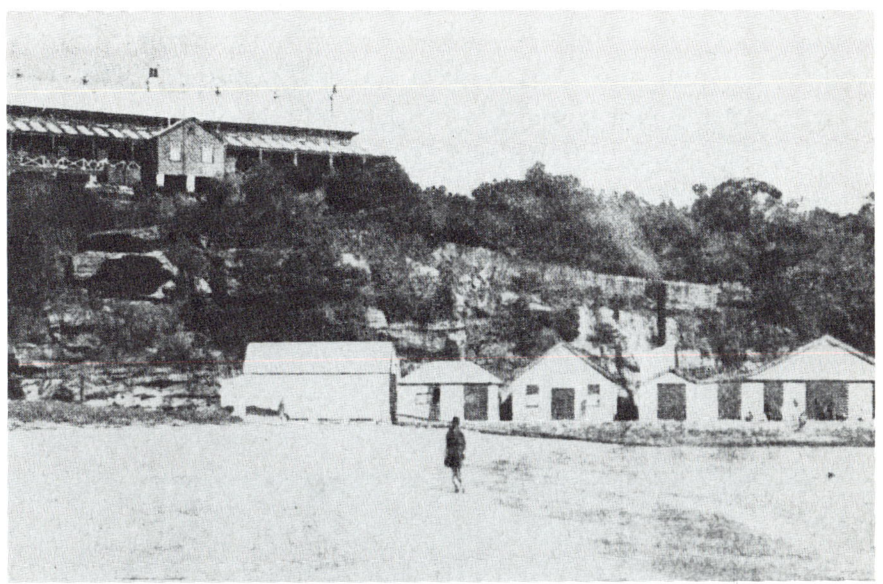

Wharf buildings and main quarantine quarters, Quarantine Station, North Head. Sydney Mail, ***31 March 1900. From the original in the General Reference Library, State Library of New South Wales***

CLEANSING AND SCAVENGING

From the outset it was clear to the authorities that the focus of the epidemic lay in and around the Darling Harbour wharves. As early as mid-February the government considered evacuating this whole area but ultimately rejected the suggestion because such a move would have been too disruptive to the colony's economy. As a compromise the health authorities urged all owners of property within the area to carry out their own intensive programme of cleansing and fumigation. Unfortunately their advice was ignored, and, as a result, late in March the government made the decision to quarantine large sections of the wharf area and undertake a programme of cleansing and rubbish removal. In the ensuing weeks the system of quarantine was extended to include large tracts of the City of Sydney and parts of Paddington, Glebe and Manly. By the conclusion of the epidemic a large proportion of Sydney's central residential and business area had been quarantined and cleansed (see Figure 63).

Once declared plague infected, streets were barricaded and right of entry and egress restricted for up to a week. Occupants were given the choice of cleansing and fumigating their own dwellings but largely such work was carried out by an official gang of cleansers, scavengers, sanitary inspectors and common labourers who descended upon each quarantined area and moved from house to house sweeping, disinfecting, limewashing, demolishing and removing large amounts of household and business rubbish. The official instructions to such teams provide some idea of the intensive nature of the undertaking. All ceilings and walls had

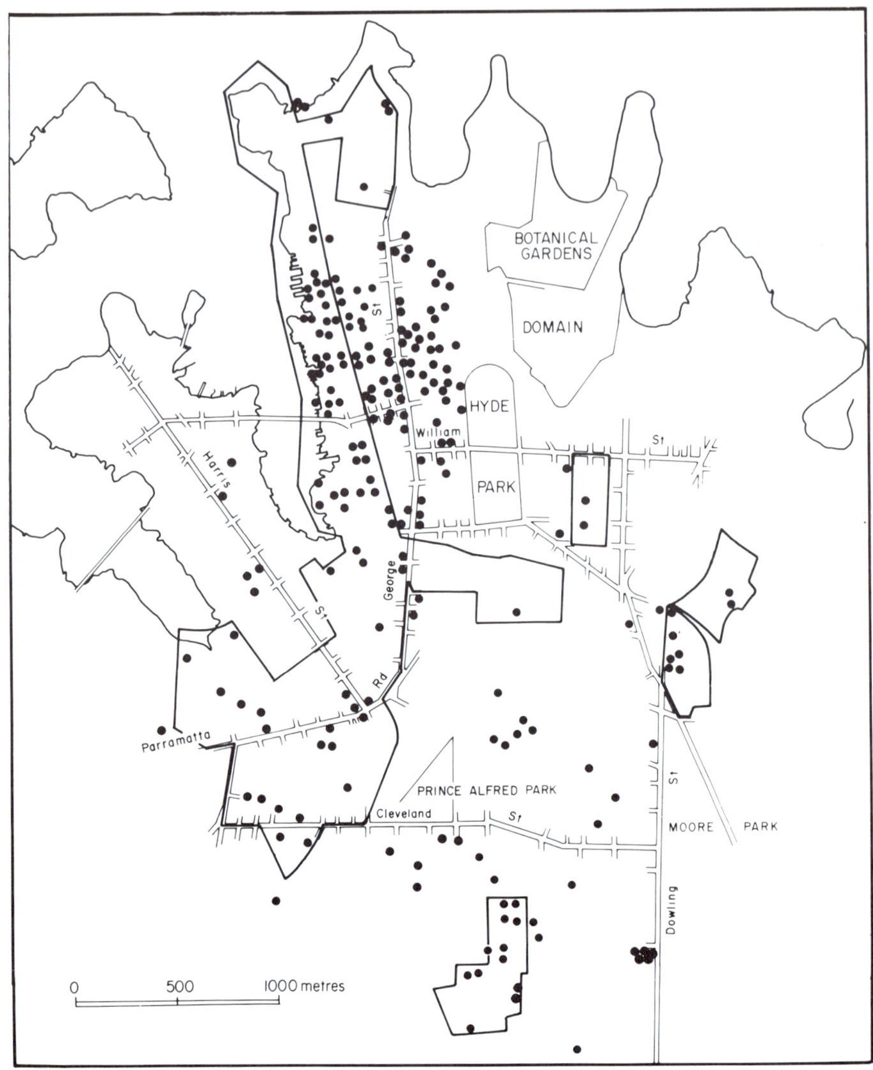

Figure 63 Plague cases and area officially cleansed 1900 (heavy lines)

to be limewashed as well as cellars and basements. All exposed woodwork was to be swabbed down with carbolic water. All floor coverings were to be removed and the floors scrubbed and swabbed with carbolic solution. Stone and brick floors inside and out were to be thoroughly saturated. All waste material, ashes and dung were to be removed. All drains, sinks and water-closets were to be flushed with hot water followed by carbolic and chloride of lime. In warehouses and business premises all merchandise was to be moved to give access to walls and floor so that they might be thoroughly cleansed as above. All buildings in bad repair were to be demolished. At the completion of these activities the occupants of the

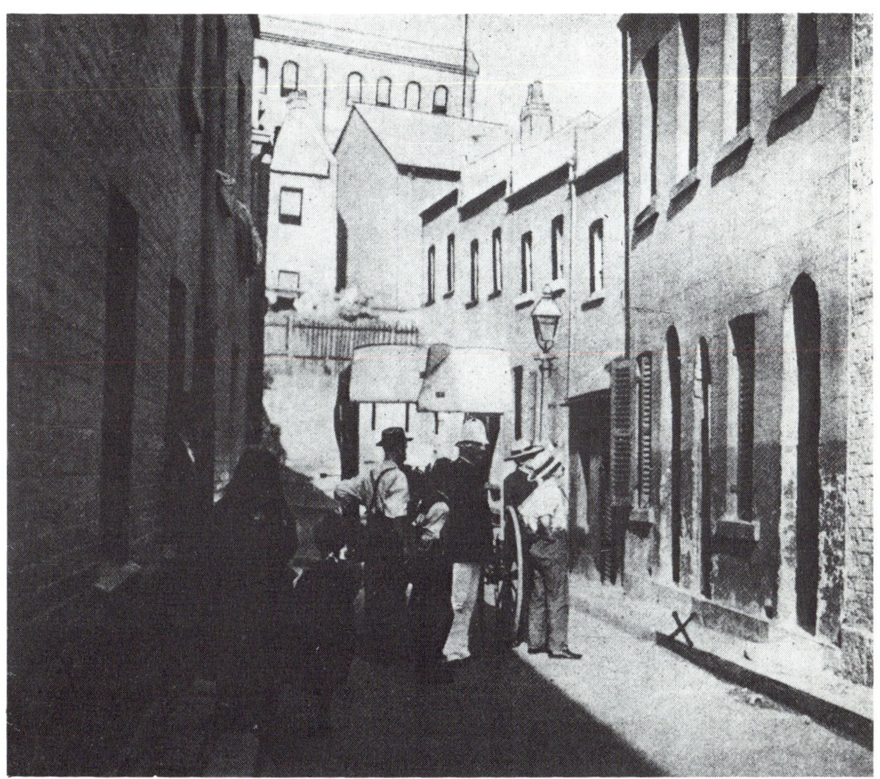

The arrival of Board of Health officers and an ambulance to remove a suspected case of plague from Bates Lane, Sussex Street in 1900.
Town and Country Journal, ***31 March 1900, p. 22. From the original in the General Reference Library, State Library of New South Wales***

cleansed premises were issued with a small placard which was to be affixed to the outside of the house. The placard stated that the dwelling had been officially cleansed of the plague infection. Such notices became for many a badge of shame and for others a signpost of areas to be strictly avoided. At any one time during the epidemic there were approximately 3000 men involved in cleansing operations in central Sydney. Their activities usually attracted a large crowd and watching their progress became for a while one of the city's major recreational pursuits. In a little over two months almost 4000 premises were formally inspected and cleansed and many thousands of tons of rubbish and filth removed.

EXTERMINATION OF RATS

One of the most important measures taken to combat the epidemic was a systematic campaign to exterminate Sydney's rodent population. A permanent gang of rat-catchers was employed in laying baits, trapping, digging out burrows and destroying the habitual haunts of rats. The Sydney City Council also employed a

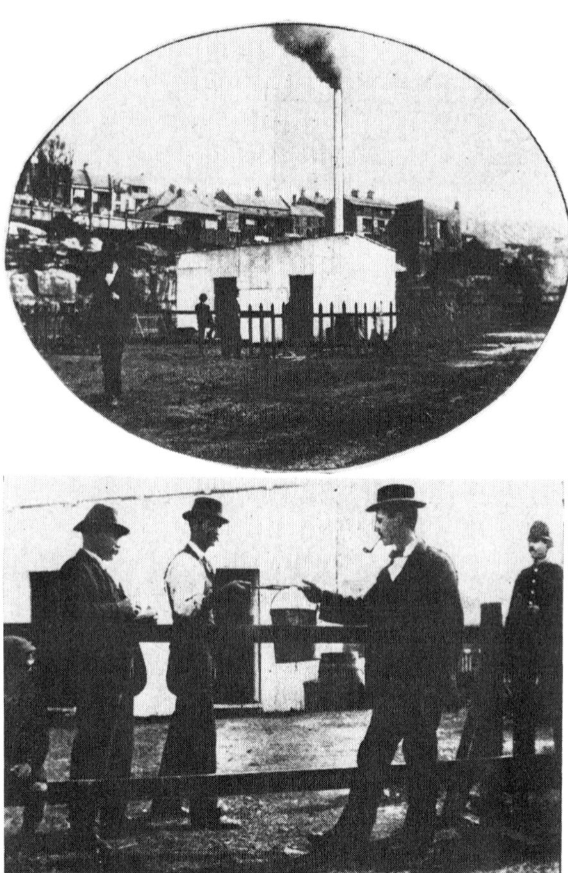

Top **The rat crematory at Darling Harbour;** ***bottom*** **Receiving rats at the crematory. Town and Country Journal,** ***31 March 1900. From the original in the General Reference Library, State Library of New South Wales***

special rat-catching squad who destroyed 38 600 rats before relinquishing their job to the official government team. In an effort to encourage people to destroy rats the government set a capitation fee of 2d. (subsequently increased to 6d.) for each rat brought in and transferred to the central depot for destruction. Between mid-April and the end of October the official rat-catchers were responsible for destroying almost 70 000 rats and if this total is added to that of the city and suburban councils' efforts then the grand total of rats killed during these months increases to more than 108 000. Early in April the Water Board began fumigating and disinfecting the city's sewage system. The effects were so dramatic as to kill many of the fish in Darling Harbour and to drive many rats away from their familiar haunts near the wharves. In retrospect the rat-extermination campaign provided some of the more humorous moments of the epidemic. There were many exotic suggestions for ridding the city of its rats, ranging from digging huge trenches and filling them with sugar to introducing ferrets to control the rat population.

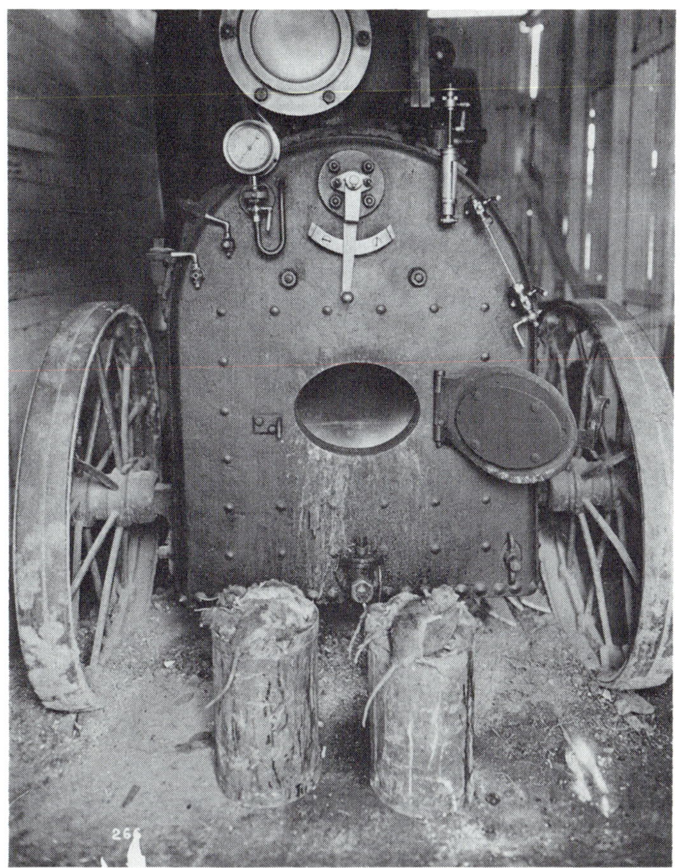

The rat incinerator.
McCreadie File, Mitchell Library, Sydney

VACCINATION

Throughout the epidemic no real effort was made to vaccinate other than those most at risk from the disease. This included not only actual cases of plague but also contacts and all medical staff. In addition, after May arrangements were made to inoculate all public servants.

The only offer of vaccination extended to the public at large occurred in the third week of March when new stocks of vaccine became available and such was the demand that supplies were quickly exhausted. On 21 March a huge throng of people suddenly arrived at the Board of Health offices demanding vaccination. In the ensuing mêlée the crowd took possession of the offices, destroyed property and forced the abandonment of the inoculation programme. The next day the government announced that vaccination would now be carried out from the Exhibition Building and strenuous efforts were made to restrict entry to those most at risk. In only a few days more than 8000 vaccinations were carried out. Soon after,

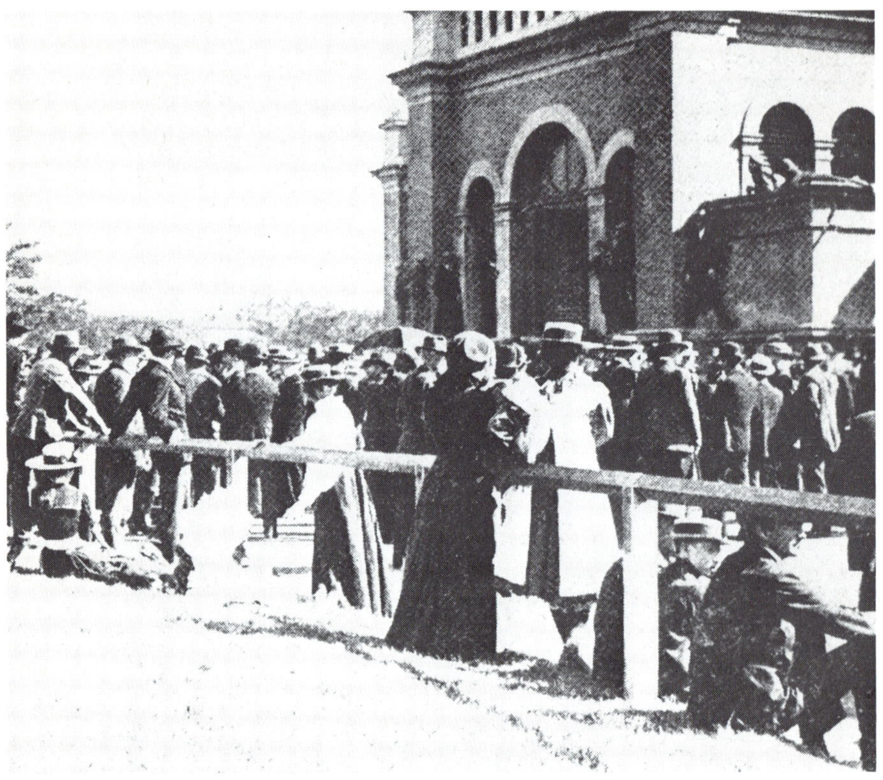

Part of the crowd waiting to be inoculated against plague in March 1900. Note the people on windowsills and ledges.
Sydney Mail, *31 March 1900, p. 752. From the original in the General Reference Library, State Library of New South Wales*

supplies of the vaccine were again depleted. Vaccination was not resumed until 11 May and in the following five weeks an additional 2700 people were vaccinated. Yersin-Roux serum became available early in May but was only administered to actual cases of plague at the Quarantine Station. From May the government continued to give preference to those persons resident or employed within the infected area. Applicants were given a dated ticket entitling them to be inoculated on a specific date.

PANIC!

Despite the small number of cases and deaths the epidemic had much in common with earlier outbreaks of plague. It caused wave after wave of horror, fear and panic to sweep through the city. The horror stemmed in large part from the centuries-old fear of plague but was undoubtedly fanned by the newspapers' reporting of the epidemic. The daily papers were full of lurid descriptions of 'The Black Death' as well as countless articles by medical 'specialists'. The papers also

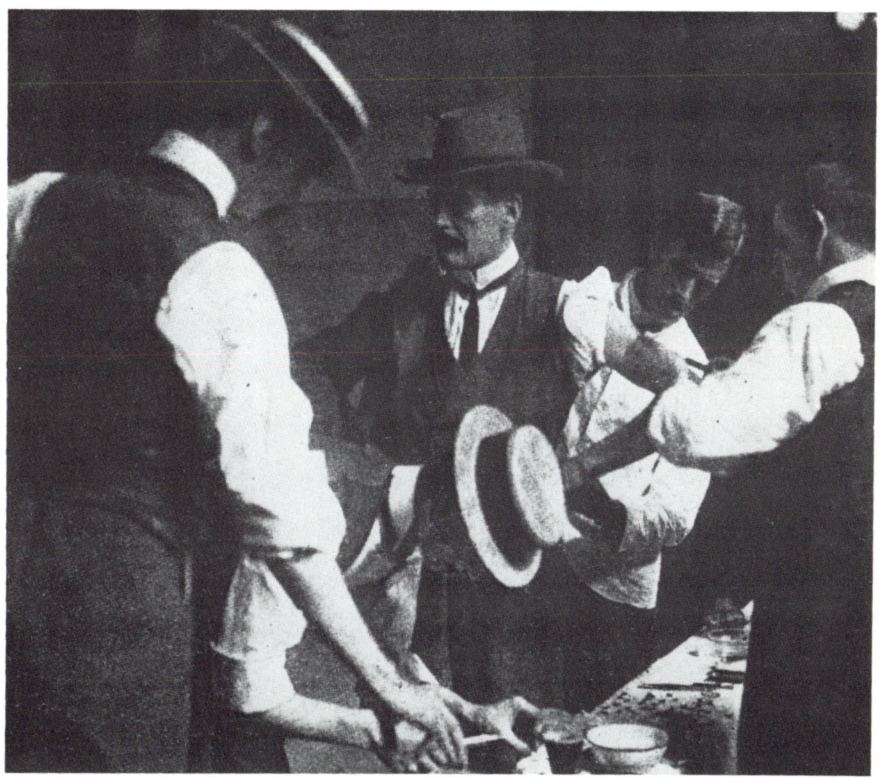

Plague contacts being inoculated during the 1900 epidemic.
Town and Country Journal, *31 March 1900. From the original in the General Reference Library, State Library of New South Wales*

carried day-to-day reports of the progress of the epidemic, including lists of its latest victims, their addresses, the fate of earlier patients, the location of quarantined premises, as well as vivid accounts of earlier plagues and the fearful mortality that they provoked. The papers were also full of charges against Sydney's Chinese community, claiming that they were responsible for introducing the disease and for hiding away those of their number who caught the plague. Add all this to the widely publicized method of burying the people who died of the plague — their bodies were wrapped in a sheet wet with sublimate solution, the lid of the coffin was screwed down, the coffin was enveloped in a coarse cloth wet with sublimate solution and buried at least 50 feet down in sandy soil on a steep slope falling to cliffs above the Pacific Ocean — and there is little doubt why panic reigned supreme.

Despite appeals to the contrary, people continued to believe that the disease was spread by personal contact. Such beliefs coloured behaviour. Shops and businesses in the quarantined areas were vigorously boycotted. The Chinese, who controlled most of the city's carpentry and joinery industry, were scrupulously avoided. When it was suspected that Sydney's fish were somehow implicated in spreading the

PUBLIC NOTICE.

BUBONIC PLAGUE.

You need not run away to the country if you take a drink of

MIGHTY "ALOK,"

WITH SODA WATER, EVERY MORNING.
MIGHTY "ALOK" fortifies the system, BUILDS up the BLOOD, and strengthens the NERVES.

IT SAVES DOCTOR'S BILLS.

It is a Refreshing, Sustaining, Stimulating TONIC, without intoxicating.
THE MOST SUCCESSFUL TONIC OF MODERN TIMES.
Ask for it in the usual or extra bitter form.
Every Hotel, with Sodawater, 6d per glass.
ALL CHEMISTS and STORES, 2/6 and 4/6 per bottle.
When being served insist upon being shown the bottle bearing our Trade Mark,

"ALOK."

Whether it be in the usual or extra bitter form the word "ALOK" must appear for you to get the GENUINE ARTICLE.

WHOLESALE AGENTS: Elliott Bros., Ltd., Australian Drug Co., Tooth and Co., J. T. and J. Toohey, Resch's Waverley Brewery, Cornwall's Australian Brewing Co., and all Wine and Spirit Merchants; also from Anthony Hordern and Sons, W. H. Soul and Co., Pattinson and Co., and Civil Service Co-operative Society.

The Talk of the Town. The Drink of the Season.
Unintoxicating.

It is an unequalled Remedy for all Stomach Complaints. A little taken every morning with Sodawater keeps the Brain, Liver, and Kidneys in perfect order.

Scientific Examination of Mighty "ALOK" by the most Eminent Authority in Australia.

Messrs. FISHER and CO. 8 Bridge-st., Sydney, February 1, 1898.
Gentlemen,—I have examined your preparation, Mighty "ALOK," and find that it contains, besides Kola Nut, only pure vegetable drugs having well-known Tonic properties.—Yours faithfully, A. HELMS.
GUARANTEED NOT TO CONTAIN QUININE OR IRON, OR ANY INJURIOUS INGREDIENT.

SOLE PROPRIETORS AND MANUFACTURERS,

FISHER & COMPANY,

PHARMACY: 337 GEORGE-STREET, NEARLY OPP. G.P.O.

The manufacturers of patent medicines and popular tonics were quick to appreciate the commercial opportunities offered by bubonic plague. Evening News, *19 March 1900, p. 8. From the original in the General Reference Library, State Library of New South Wales*

disease people boycotted the city's fish dealers and Cardinal Moran declared that the faithful could eat meat during Lent.[3] People avoided dwellings and streets from where plague victims had been removed, reported on those suspected of being ill or hiding plague cases and agitated for the quarantine of others. Typical of this sort of reaction was a letter received by the Board of Health early in April from a group of city merchants calling for the removal and quarantine of a York Street undertaker simply because he was involved in removing the bodies of plague victims. At a more general level the newspapers were full of stories of people stampeding to leave Sydney either for the suburbs or for the Blue Mountains. Of

[3] Most of the fish around the Darling Harbour and the Central wharves died as a result of the outfall of disinfectants and fumigants poured into the city's drains and sewers. In the popular mind the fish died from bubonic plague (see the *Bulletin*, 31 March 1900:10).

THE PLAGUE.

Owing to the scare caused by the Plague, numbers of families have kept away from the city, and visitors from the country and adjoining colonies have been conspicuous by their absence. The consequence to trade is that there is a surplusage in our stocks of winter articles, especially of high-class qualities. There are two ways of dealing with such surplus stock—packing it away for next winter, or turning it into ready money at cost price, or under, at once. We prefer this latter method, and have, therefore, decided while the cold weather is still to come, to give our customers the benefit, by holding a Special

MIDWINTER SALE,

when all our Winter Stock will be offered at a little over cost price, and in many instances, where our stocks are too large, such as in Ladies' Travelling Cloaks, Furs, Coats, and Skirts, Wool Wraps, Blankets, Dress Materials, Flannelettes, etc., our prices will be below cost.

This Great Midwinter Sale commences on THURSDAY MORNING.

The Mutual Stores will be closed all day TODAY (WEDNESDAY), to enable us to unpack and re-mark goods which MUST BE SOLD during this Special Sale.

THE MUTUAL STORES,

PITT-STREET,

Next Door to the Strand Arcade.

By mid-1900 most of Sydney's business houses were including mention of plague in their regular advertisements.
Evening News, *30 May 1900, p. 8. From the original in the General Reference Library, State Library of New South Wales*

the general reaction Billy Hughes was later to write: 'we must remember that there was a panic — that every man, or nearly every man, who could afford it left Sydney — that thousands of visitors who were coming here avoided Sydney as if it were leprous' (Hughes, 1900:208).

Plague was viewed by many as an expression of God's wrath at man's sinfulness and the churches appealed for divine intervention. At the height of the epidemic Sydney's churches set aside a Day of Humiliation and Prayer and from all accounts most churches were crowded to overflowing. The alarm and confusion generated by the epidemic spread well beyond Sydney and New South Wales. Most of the other Australian colonies instituted vigorous precautions against goods and passenger services from New South Wales and in New Zealand the postal authorities formally insisted that all mail from New South Wales be fumigated. The epidemic also caused serious disruption to the shipping services between Australia and New Zealand. The decline in passenger traffic and the frequent delays due to the

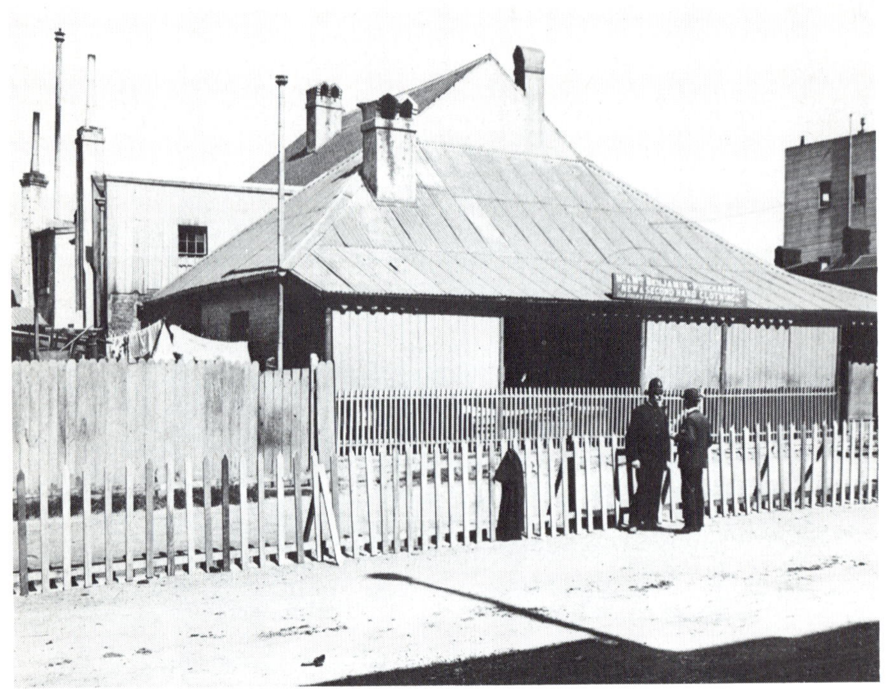

109 Goulburn Street showing the official quarantine line. 'Infected' premises and their immediate neighbours were barricaded off from the street, a police guard was mounted and the public warned to keep away.
McCreadie File, Mitchell Library, Sydney

enforcement of quarantine procedures caused great financial loss to the Union Steamship Company (Maclean, 1964:283).

Although panic gripped many of Sydney's inhabitants from late March until well into June the public contribution in helping bring the epidemic under control was not insignificant. Local Sanitary Committees were organized in a number of municipalities and in April a Citizen's Vigilance Committee with branches throughout the city was established. Largely these *ad hoc* bodies were set up to monitor local public health and sanitary conditions and to enlist local householders in rat-killing. The Vigilance Committee frequently lobbied the government and Board of Health, such as when they complained about rat-catchers being permitted to transport their catch aboard the city's trams to the downtown furnaces.

Against the rising tide of panic there were a few isolated voices which called for calm and a measured assessment of the epidemic. The *Bulletin*, for example, somewhat more restrained in its reporting of the epidemic than most of Sydney's papers and journals, wrote in late March:

So far the plague . . . is a very small affair. It isn't a patch on the daily, hourly typhoid as a means of slaughtering the public, and so far it has proved about as safe as football, and much safer than it was a few weeks ago to have doubts concerning the absolute justice of the war in South Africa. (*Bulletin*, 31 March 1900:6)

All this was undoubtedly true. Compared with the annual death toll in the city from scarlet fever, diphtheria, typhoid and consumption, plague was only a relatively 'small affair'. Yet that is not how most of the people saw it. They shied away in horror from the disease.

POPULAR CURES

The epidemic gave the manufacturers and purveyors of patent medicines and quack cures a bonanza. The rapidity with which such people appreciated the commercial possibilities of the outbreak was demonstrated by the fact that the first popular advertisement referring to plague appeared as early as 17 January, two days before any cases of plague had been declared in Sydney. This advertisement followed the report of possible plague cases in Adelaide and like most of those that followed was clearly designed to foster public concern. The produce advertised was Vitadatio, one of the 'great' herbal remedies of the late nineteenth century. Not to be outdone the manufacturers of Dr Morse's Indian Root Pills, Bile Beans, Mighty Alok, Alfaline Herbal Remedies and countless others quickly followed suit. Most advertisers played on past fears and quoted in highly emotive language grim reminders of past epidemics and man's inability to cope with such outbreaks. By late March the warnings began to take a more sinister and ominous note, quoting the number of deaths and cases quarantined and referring to the widespread consternation in the city. Most advertisements were full of dire warnings, of reminders of past epidemics, of the need for personal vigilance, and played on human frailties and anxieties. By mid-April not only were the purveyors of popular medicines having a field-day but their ranks had also been joined by many general retailers and manufacturers of a large variety of household goods, insurance agents and real estate companies. From this date Sydney's newspapers were full of advertisements recommending anti-plague cures, a wide range of disinfectants and fumigating agents, cigarettes, tonic waters, clothing, eucalyptus oil, etc. Even insurance agents added bubonic plague to their list of insurable calamities, for example the First Accident Company which provided £12 per week during disablement from bubonic plague, typhus, diphtheria, smallpox, typhoid, scarlet fever and measles. At the height of the epidemic one real estate company was canvassing suburban properties on the basis that they were located well away from the area affected by plague. In early April Vitadatio even ran an open letter to the people of Sydney offering to pay £10 to the first person to catch plague while taking their product. No takers came forward.

CONCLUSIONS

The last case of plague occurred on 2 August and the last death some two weeks later. Sydney breathed a heavy sigh of relief. But the relief was to be short-lived. Plague was to break out again a year later and was to remain a threat for at least the next ten years. In the end the 1900 epidemic was a great social calamity which

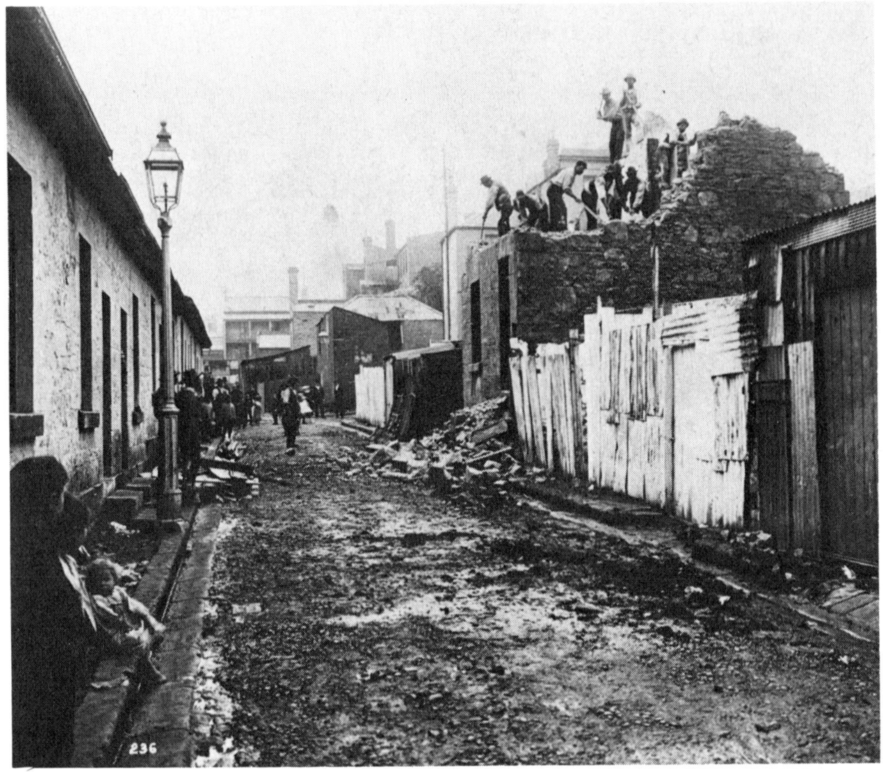

Watched by local residents a team of workmen demolish an infected property in Johnstone's Lane during the plague epidemic. Note that the adjoining fences have been limewashed.
McCreadie File, Mitchell Library, Sydney

produced considerable social and economic disruption. To some, however, it was a blessing in disguise for it served to draw attention to the insanitary and depressed living conditions of many city dwellers and to the fact that Sydney was an ill-regulated and ill-governed city. It also led to the resumption and remodelling of the Darling Harbour wharves and adjacent area and to increasing pressure for sanitary, health and local government reform.

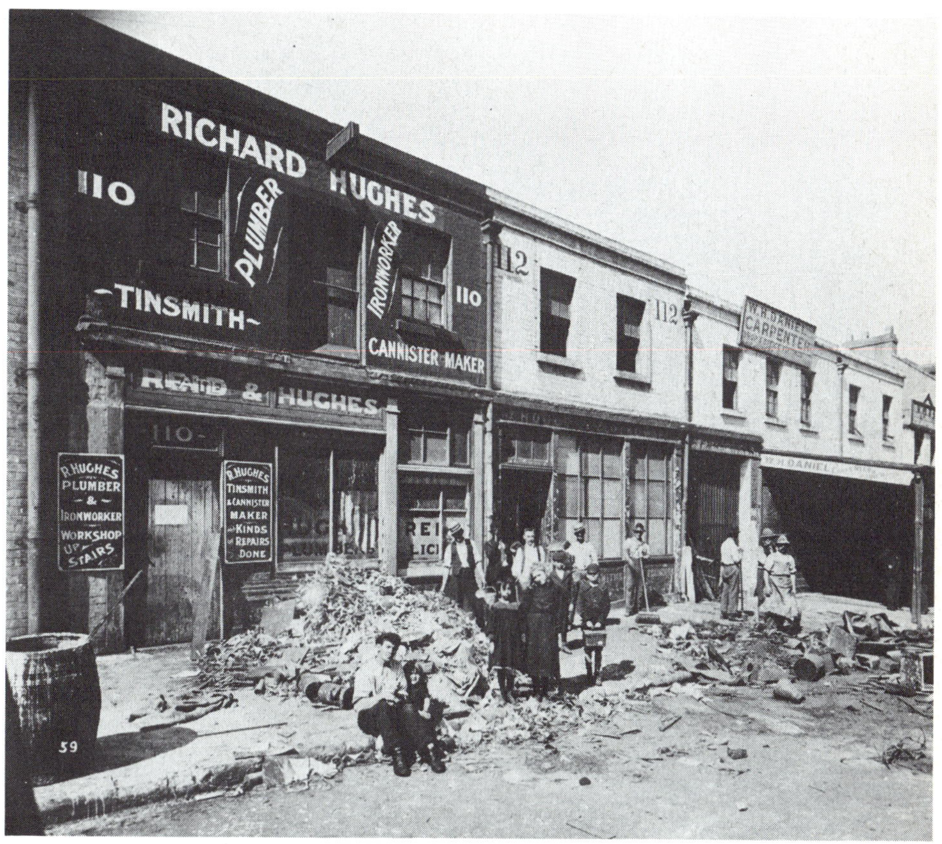

A group of small businesses in Sussex Street at the time of the plague clean-up in 1900. Most rubbish was dumped on the streetside to await collection. Note the barrel of limewash used to coat exterior walls and floors.
McCreadie File, Mitchell Library, Sydney

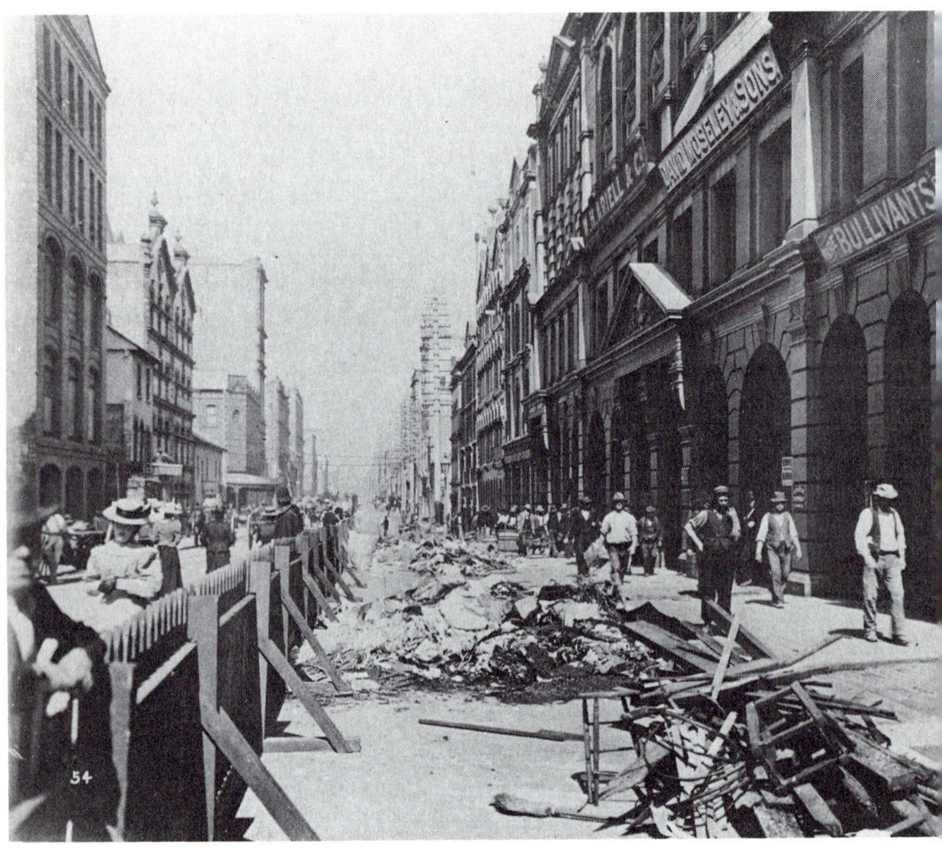

Kent Street at the height of the plague epidemic. The official barrier and police guard served to segregate plague workers and sanitary teams from the general public.
McCreadie File, Mitchell Library, Sydney

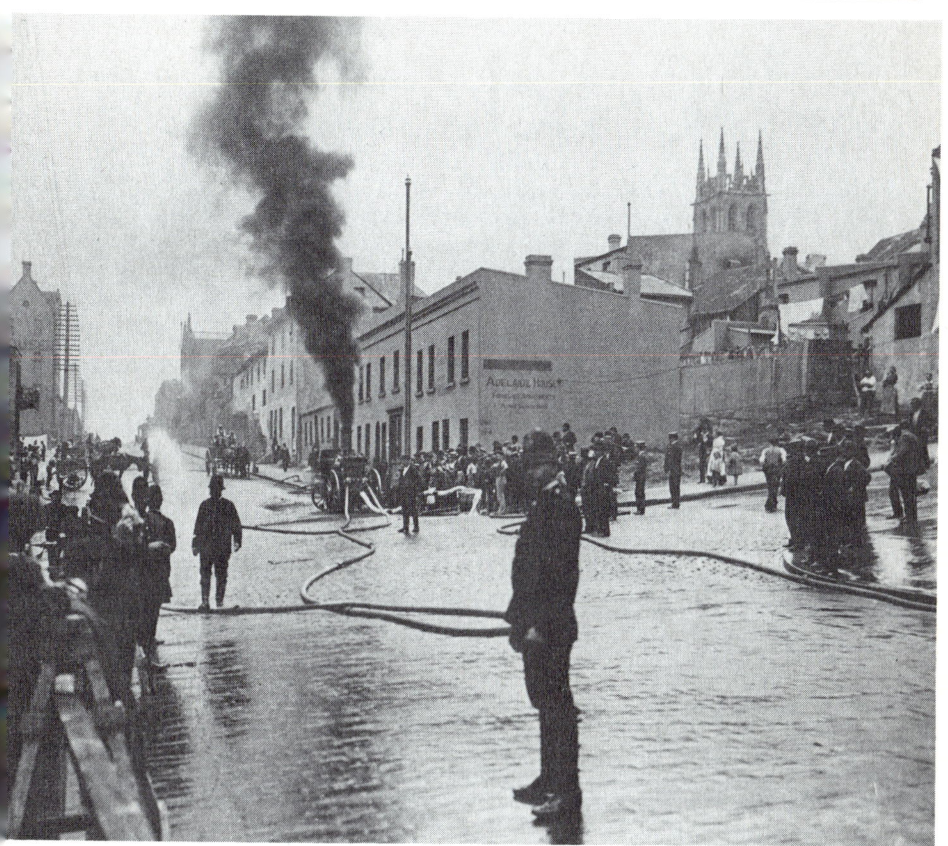

Cleansing Sydney's street during the plague outbreak in 1900. During the epidemic teams of scavengers and cleansers systematically worked their way through Sydney's central residential and business districts.
McCreadie File, Mitchell Library, Sydney

CHAPTER NINE

Conclusions

Epidemics of infectious disease were a familiar and inescapable feature of nineteenth-century Sydney life, a regular reminder of the insecurity of life and the ubiquitous presence of death and disease. Although such epidemics were usually short-lived and for the most part not great demographic crises they none the less remained memorable events and their effects were wide-ranging. To the majority of Sydney's population they were unpredictable acts of fate, an expression of God's wrath. They were also seen as a symptom of disorder in the universe and a natural consequence of cosmic disturbance and personal excess. Although all had their origin outside Australia they were not wholly independent of local social and economic conditions. Overcrowding, poor housing, lack of sanitation, and polluted water all served to determine the local incidence and severity of epidemic disease.

In general, epidemics carried off the least resistant members of the population and during the nineteenth century that normally meant the lower classes. Rarely were members of the middle and upper classes affected. Poverty, malnutrition and disease went hand in hand. In many ways the history of epidemic disease and premature death in Sydney is the history of the poor. Most of the epidemics in this book reveal this only too well. Even in the case of measles in 1867 and influenza in 1891, when infection was fairly widespread, it was Sydney's most disadvantaged groups that still bore the heaviest burden. If epidemic disease had a social dimension it also had a spatial manifestation as well. The centralized location of Sydney's poor and disadvantaged groups meant that infectious disease was spatially concentrated, and even when the poor residential areas expanded into Woolloomooloo, Surry Hills and Ultimo, disease accompanied the residential shift. In spatial terms, therefore, the history of epidemic disease is one of bouts of infection sweeping through particular residential areas time after time. The Rocks, the residential area adjacent to Darling Harbour, Pyrmont, Woolloomooloo, Surry Hills, Waterloo and Botany were the loci of infectious disease throughout the nineteenth century. Yet it was not always only where a person lived that determined his or her susceptibility to infectious disease. The 1900 plague epidemic shows only too well the importance of place of work and how infection could be closely tied to the economic structure of the city.

What distinguished these epidemics from the many other perils of nineteenth-century life was not so much the danger of the diseases themselves as the extraordinary and often severe measures advanced for their control. Ill-conceived and hastily organized policies of quarantine, isolation, cleansing, scavenging and medical treatment were partly responsible for the upsurge of emotional reaction that accompanied the passage of each epidemic. Moreover, the impact of these measures fell mainly upon Sydney's lower classes who were the real victims of the piece. Their lives were imperilled, their movement restricted, their homes demolished or ill-treated and their possessions scattered. These official measures were greeted by fear, resentment and anger. Unlike Sydney's upper classes few options existed to the poor other than prayers, obedience or flight.

These epidemics like all traumatic experiences accentuated the worst in Sydney at the time. They highlighted the inadequacies and deficiencies in public health and government, neither of which could cope with an unfamiliar and sudden disaster with the means at their disposal. Prior to 1881 no administrative structure existed for dealing with indigenous cases of infectious disease, there was no special isolation hospital, and the only regulations available were those specifically dealing with maritime quarantine which were more honoured in the breach than in the observance. Some centralized public health authority was clearly necessary and the Board of Health which appeared as a result of the smallpox outbreak in 1881–2 ushered in a new era of public health. Dealing with epidemics also called for co-operation between the central authority and local government bodies as well as a clear philosophy regarding public health. Even after 1881 the Board of Health had to struggle against self-interest, ignorance, panic and over-reaction. The over-zealous policy of quarantine, whereby many people were incarcerated for no apparent reason, produced many examples of personal and family tragedy and business ruin.

These epidemics also served to expose gross social evils. They drew attention to the housing and living conditions of Sydney's poor and the inadequacies of sanitation and public hygiene. Towards the end of the century they also stirred the conscience of Sydney's middle class and led to a movement for sanitary reform.

Disease has numerous effects: demographic, social, economic, medical, geographical and psychological. Any great crisis inevitably leaves its mark on the attitudes and behaviour of the group. These epidemics were no exception. With the exception of the measles outbreak in 1867, all caused an immense emotional reaction and an upsurge of anxiety and despair to sweep through Sydney. In this sense the psychological repercussions far outweighed the demographic. For many people these epidemics were shattering personal experiences and the feeling of helpless exposure produced widespread demoralization and despair. In places this reached the level of mass hysteria and panic. Possibly the general emotion and anxiety surrounding a particular epidemic served to mould the attitudes and behaviour of subsequent generations and, if this was so, then our attitude towards disease today owes much to the reaction and behaviour of our forebears. One basic problem that remains unresolved concerns the reactions of the poor to these periodic disasters. No record exists as to how they felt or reacted, or how their lives were transformed by the loss of children, husbands, wives or other close relatives. It was not the poor who wrote letters to the newspapers or the Board of Health or who joined the Health Society or Sanitary Committees. Did they, as Eversley suggests, stoically and uncomplainingly bear the personal devastation and tragedy of repeated waves of disease and premature death? How did disease affect their fertility and home life? Did widows/widowers quickly remarry? Did the effects of such outbreaks remain indelibly etched on their memories? Regrettably the record is silent on such matters.

Anxiety and fear brought into the open old tensions and antagonisms. The search for scapegoats resulted in a virulent anti-Chinese campaign which was possibly orchestrated by certain politicians with a view to ending Chinese immigration. While these disasters reinforced existing prejudice against the Chinese they also gave rise to a series of social conflicts — neighbour against neighbour, merchant against merchant, anti-vaccinators against pro-vaccinators, doctor against doctor, central government versus local government. In all this the press played a vital role. The newspapers did little to create an environment of calm. The instinct to play on people's fears proved irresistible and there is little doubt that the press helped spread wild hysterical rumours. The newspapers also fed the public's appetite for popular cures and undoubtedly added an air of legitimacy to the claims of many manufacturers of popular cures and quack medicines. Many in the business community saw these epidemics as a way of increasing profits. Publicans peddled their stocks of 'anti-plague ales', chemists their wide range of disinfectants and fumigants, while the makers of Dr Morse's Indian Root Pills, Mighty Alok and Vitadatio invented even more extravagant claims. The feverish desire with which the public embraced such popular cures tells us something about the status and role of formal medicine and the need for people to seek resort in traditional folk and popular cures during times of severe crisis.

The social and economic impact of these six epidemics varied considerably. There is no denying the major impact of the 1789 crisis on Aboriginal society, although whether the effects were as long-lasting or as widespread as later generations have come to believe is disputable. The epidemics that caused the most disruption to the city and affected the lives of most Sydney dwellers all occurred during the last twenty years of the century. The outbreaks of smallpox, influenza and bubonic plague, partly because of the historical fear of such pestilences, caused major disruption to Sydney's everyday life. Of the three, only the influenza outbreak of 1891 incapacitated large numbers of the population. The other two in terms of their epidemiological impact were relatively minor affairs. Yet both produced incredible scenes of community disruption, paralysed much of the city's normal social and business activities and resulted in draconian measures of control.

This study began with the observation that there were two distinctive types of epidemic crisis, one differentiated in terms of the high morbidity and mortality produced within a restricted time-space framework, the other by the psychosocial reaction produced. One of the ironies of Sydney's nineteenth-century epidemiological history is that the epidemics that produced the highest mortality (measles and scarlet fever) largely engendered the least public reaction. By comparison, the outbreaks of smallpox and bubonic plague, although less significant in terms of cases and deaths, produced the greatest scenes of hysteria, fear and social disruption. These epidemics also made a much more vivid impression on those who lived through them. In many cases they left enduring memories and became part of popular history. Some, like the 1789 'smallpox' outbreak, could even grow in the memory over the years and eventually assume larger-than-life proportions.

These epidemics demand attention for a number of reasons. In the first place, they were a prime cause of public health reform. In the second, they represent striking evidence of the insanitary and impoverished living conditions of Sydney's working classes in the nineteenth century. In the third, they put to the test and challenged colonial comprehension and management of extreme natural events. Finally, they throw into sharp perspective the internal workings and tensions of colonial society.

The study of the impact, diffusion and effects of historical epidemics is a rewarding experience from a number of points of view. Firstly, there is a need for retrospective studies of the behaviour of epidemics in different populations exposed to a variety of health care circumstances. Secondly, close observation of the way people and communities behave during times of severe stress and crisis can reveal a great deal about social attitudes, patterns of activity, interaction and mobility, underlying tensions and antagonisms, as well as many other aspects which may not be readily apparent under more normal circumstances. Thirdly, the experience of such catastrophes may result in significant changes in community values, attitudes and behaviour. Finally, in the words of Michael Roe, such crises 'served the supreme purpose of the local historian: to gain some sense of how our fellows — in [time and] space met the challenge of life and death' (Roe, 1976:145).

Appendix One

Temporal Schedule of Epidemics

Measles 1867

Week	
1	6–12 February
2	13–19 February
3	20–26 February
4	27 February–5 March
5	6–12 March
6	13–19 March
7	20–26 March
8	27 March–2 April
9	3–9 April
10	10–16 April
11	17–23 April
12	24–30 April
13	1–7 May
14	8–14 May
15	15–21 May
16	22–28 May
17	29 May–4 June
18	5–11 June
19	12–18 June
20	19–25 June
21	26 June–2 July
22	3–9 July
23	10–16 July
24	17–23 July
25	24–30 July

Scarlet Fever 1875–6

Week	
1	28 September–4 October
2	5–11 October
3	12–18 October
4	19–25 October
5	26 October–1 November
6	2–8 November
7	9–15 November
8	16–22 November
9	23–29 November
10	30 November–6 December
11	7–13 December
12	14–20 December
13	21–27 December
14	28 December–3 January
15	4–10 January
16	11–17 January
17	18–24 January
18	25–31 January
19	1–7 February
20	8–14 February
21	15–21 February
22	22–28 February
23	29 February–6 March
24	7–13 March
25	14–20 March
26	21–27 March
27	28 March–3 April
28	4–10 April
29	11–17 April
30	18–24 April
31	25 April–1 May
32	2–8 May
33	9–15 May
34	16–22 May
35	23–29 May
36	30 May–5 June
37	6–12 June
38	13–19 June
39	20–26 June
40	27 June–3 July

Scarlet Fever 1875–6

Fortnights	
1	28 September–11 October
2	12–25 October
3	26 October–8 November
4	9–22 November
5	23 November–6 December
6	7–20 December
7	21 December–3 January
8	4–17 January
9	18–31 January
10	1–14 February
11	15–28 February
12	29 February–13 March
13	14–27 March
14	28 March–10 April
15	11–24 April
16	25 April–8 May
17	9–22 May
18	23 May–5 June
19	6–19 June
20	20 June–3 July

Smallpox 1881–2

Week	
1	25–31 May
2	1–7 June
3	8–14 June
4	15–21 June
5	22–28 June
6	29 June–5 July
7	6–12 July
8	13–19 July
9	20–26 July
10	27 July–2 August
11	3–9 August
12	10–16 August
13	17–23 August
14	24–30 August
15	31 August–6 September
16	7–13 September
17	14–20 September
18	21–27 September
19	28 September–4 October
20	5–11 October
21	12–18 October
22	19–25 October
23	26 October–1 November
24	2–8 November
25	9–15 November
26	16–22 November
27	23–29 November
28	30 November–6 December
29	7–13 December
30	14–20 December
31	21–27 December
32	28 December–3 January
33	4–10 January
34	11–17 January
35	18–24 January
36	25–31 January
37	1–7 February
38	8–14 February
39	15–21 February
40	22–28 February

APPENDIX ONE

Plague 1900

Week	
1	19–25 January
2	26 January–1 February
3	2–8 February
4	9–15 February
5	16–22 February
6	23 February–1 March
7	2–8 March
8	9–15 March
9	16–22 March
10	23–29 March
11	30 March–5 April
12	6–12 April
13	13–19 April
14	20–26 April
15	27 April–3 May
16	4–10 May
17	11–17 May
18	18–24 May
19	25–31 May
20	1–7 June
21	8–14 June
22	15–21 June
23	22–28 June
24	29 June–5 July
25	6–12 July
26	13–19 July
27	20–26 July
28	27 July–2 August
29	3–9 August
30	10–16 August

Appendix Two

Local Government Boundaries Referred to in the Text

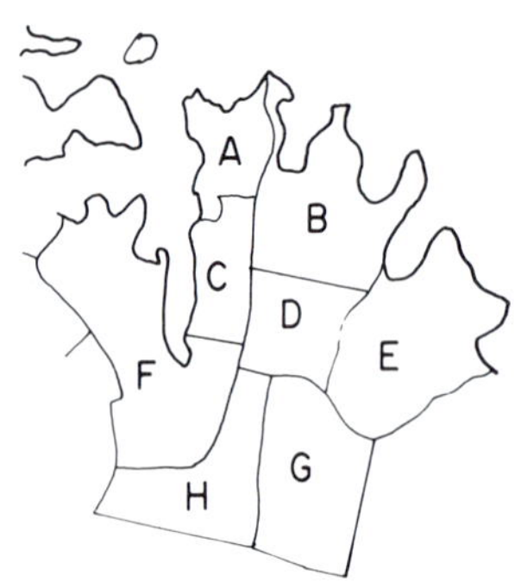

City of Sydney Wards
1867-1900

A Gipps
B Bourke
C Brisbane
D Macquarie
E Fitzroy
F Denison
G Cook
H Phillip

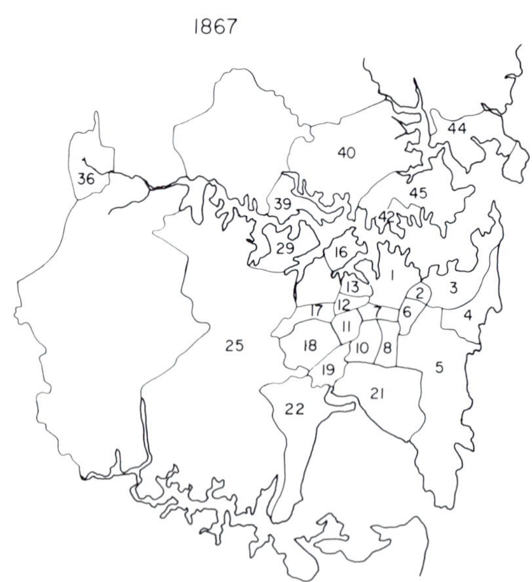

APPENDIX TWO

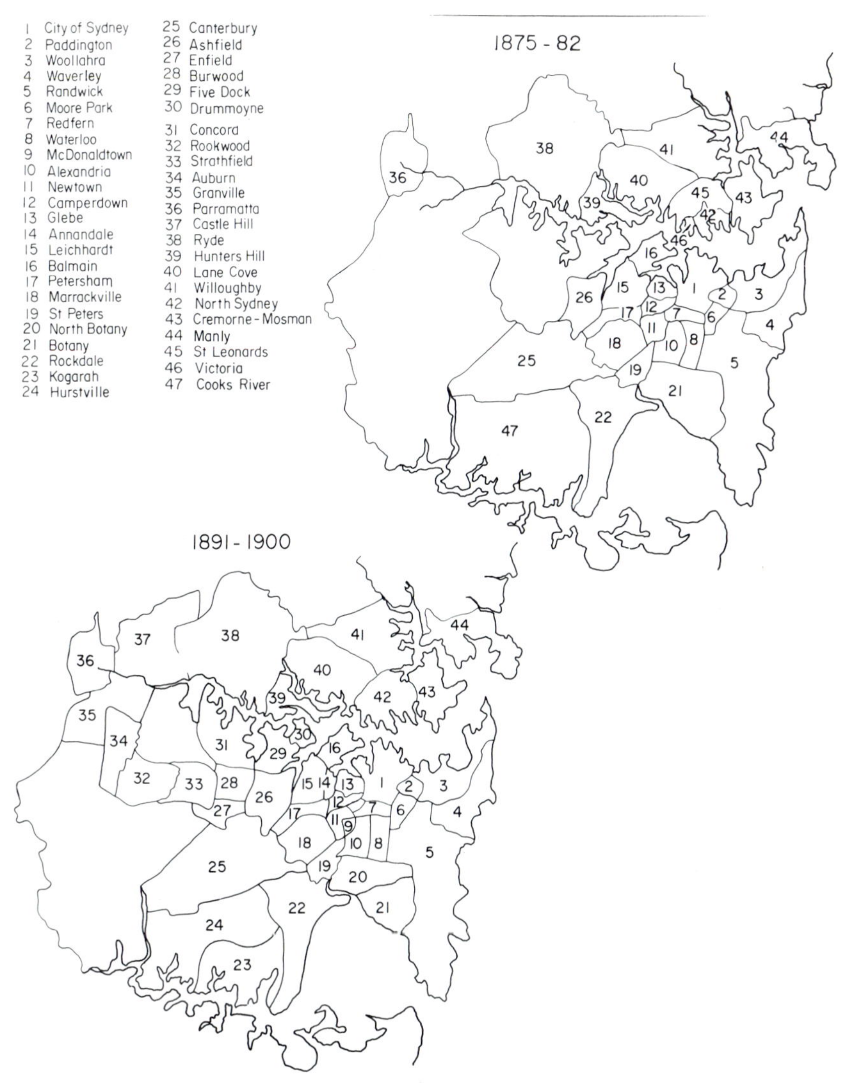

Appendix Three

Diffusion of Plague Cases by Place of Work, February–May 1900

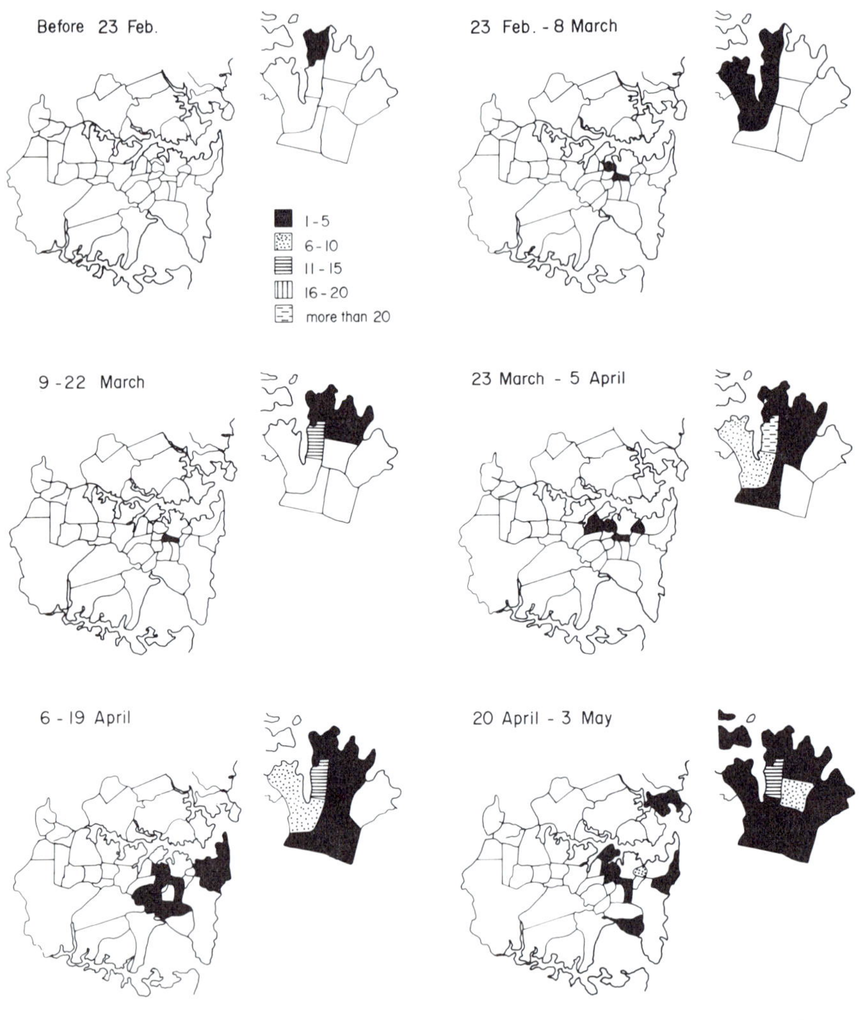

APPENDIX THREE

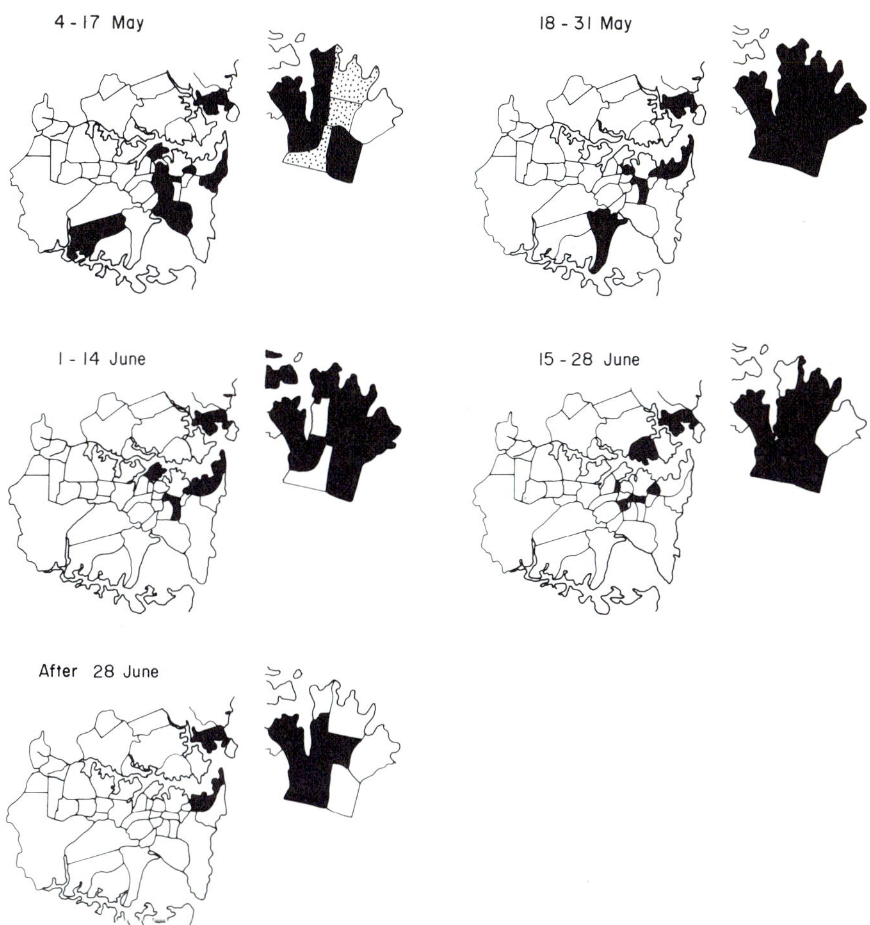

Sources of Figures

Figure	*Source*
1	*HRA* I, 2, 1914; *HRA* I, 3, 1915.
2–7	Sydney Dispensary/Infirmary, Annual Return of Diseases Treated, 1836–65.
8	Metropolitan Board of Water Supply and Sewerage, Plan of Sydney [ML].
9	Director-General of Public Health, *Annual Reports of Medical Officer of Health*, 1898–1900.
10	Parish Registers, Convict Records, 1788–1856; Registrar-General, Vital Statistics, 1857–1900; Cumpston, 1914, 1927; Cumpston and McCallum, 1927; Gandevia, 1978; Jamieson, 1908.
11–13, 18	Parish Registers, Convict Records, 1811–56; Registrar-General, Vital Statistics, 1857–1900.
14–17	Registrar-General, Vital Statistics, 1856–1900.
19	Parish Registers, Convict Records, 1841.
20	Board of Health, Map of City of Sydney with Location of Deaths 1889 [RACP].
21	Registrar-General, Vital Statistics, 1900.
22	Aboriginal 'pathways' from Ross, 1976, with permission.
23–30, 33	Registrar-General, Death Records, 1867.
32	After Morley, 1980.
34–42	Registrar-General, Death Records, 1875–6.
43	Tidswell, 1898; Cumpston, 1914.
44–49	*SMH*, 1881–2; Board of Health, 1883; Cumpston, 1914.
50, 51, 53	Ashburton-Thompson, 1892.
52, 54, 55	Registrar-General, Death Records, 1891.
56	Gladesville Asylum, *Report of the Inspector-General of the Insane 1891.*
57–62	Register of Cases of Bubonic Plague, 1900 [AO].
63	*SMH*, 1900.

References

Abbreviations

AO	Archives Office of New South Wales, Sydney
CS	Census and Statistics Library, Sydney
HC	Health Commission of New South Wales, Sydney
HRA	*Historical Records of Australia*
HRNSW	*Historical Records of New South Wales*
ML	Mitchell Library, Sydney
PRO	Public Records Office, London
RACP	Royal Australasian College of Physicians Library, Sydney
SMH	*Sydney Morning Herald*
St P	St Philips Church

A. UNPUBLISHED SOURCES

1. Parish Burial Records

(Church of England unless otherwise stated)

St Andrews, 1842–57; St Andrews (Presbyterian), 1837–56; Christchurch St Lawrence, 1838–76; Holy Trinity, 1843–58; St James, 1824–58; St Marys (Roman Catholic), 1821–58; St Philips, 1787–1860; St Thomas, 1850–60; St Lukes, 1849–57.

2. Cemetery Burial Registers

Balmain General Cemetery, 1868–82; Bridge Street (Jewish), 1846–66; Camperdown Cemetery (Church of England Burial Company), 1849–69; Petersham Cemetery (Catholic), 1865–86; Rookwood Cemetery, 1869–82; York Street and Great Synagogue (Jewish), 1867–80.

3. Registrar-General of New South Wales: Official Burial and Death Records

Alexandria Register, 1853–6; Baptist Burial Records, 1840–56; Independent Burial Records, 1841–56; Jewish Burial Records, 1831–66; Sydney Death Records, 1867, 1875–6, 1881–2, 1891, 1900; Wesleyan Burial Records, 1839–56.

4. Convict Burial Records

Convict Death Register, 1821–79 [AO]; Registration of Death and Commutation Warrants, 1821–4 [AO].

5. Sydney Hospital Records

(a) *Deaths*

Quarterly Returns of Deaths and Returns of Deaths, 1811–26. [ML]

Weekly Reports of Deaths, January–October 1826. [ML]

(b) *Disease and Treatment*
Sydney Hospital, Dispensary Book, 26 May–7 November 1808, 12–23 November 1808. [ML]
Sydney Hospital, Outpatient Record Book, 4 November 1817–2 May 1819. [ML]
Sydney Hospital, Day Book, 31 August–24 October 1819. [ML]
Sydney Hospital, Hospital Muster Books, 1830–60. Admiralty Papers [PRO]
A List of Medicines for the Use of H.M. Colony in N.S.W., 12 July 1788. [PRO]

6. Disease Records

Register of Cases of Bubonic Plague, 1900–8. [AO]

7. Other

Cummins, C.J. 1966. *The genesis and development of health services in New South Wales (1788–1855).* Dept of Public Health Report to Public Service Board, Sydney. Typescript. [HC]

———. 1971. *The development of the Benevolent (Sydney) Asylum 1788–1855.* Dept of Health, Sydney. Typescript. [HC]

———. n.d. *The administration of medical services in New South Wales 1788–1855.* Dept of Public Health, Sydney. Typescript. [HC]

Randwick Asylum for Destitute Children, Register of Inmates, 1852–76. [AO]

St Philips Parochial Register, 1882–5. [St P]

8. Thesis

Ross, A. 1976. Intertribal contacts — What the First Fleet saw. BA Hons thesis, University of Sydney.

9. Maps

Board of Health, Map of the City of Sydney with Location of Deaths from Particular Diseases for 1889. [E. Ford Collection RACP]

Metropolitan Board of Water Supply and Sewage, Plan of Sydney and Suburbs . . . Showing Reported Cases of Typhoid Fever for the Year 1894. [ML]

Sydney Metropolitan Area Municipalities 1861, 1871, 1881, 1891, 1901. [CS]

10. Newspapers and Journals

Bulletin, Sydney, 1880–1900.
Sydney Morning Herald (SMH), 1867, 1875–6, 1881–2, 1891, 1900.

B. PUBLISHED SOURCES

Alexander, J.T. 1980. *Bubonic plague in early modern Russia.* Johns Hopkins University Press, Baltimore.

Angulo, J.J., C.K. Takiguti, C.A.A. Pederneiras, A.M. Carvalho-de-Souza and M.C. Oliveira-Souza. 1979. Identification of pattern and process in the spread of a contagious disease. *Social Science and Medicine* 13D:183–9.

Ashburton-Thompson, J. 1892. *Report on epidemic of influenza during 1891.* Legislative Assembly of N.S.W. Papers, 1892–3, Vol. 3. Government Printer, Sydney.

———. 1901. *Report on outbreak of plague at Sydney 1900.* Legislative Assembly of N.S.W. Papers, 1900, Vol. 11. Government Printer, Sydney.

———. 1903. *Report of the Board of Health on a second outbreak of plague at Sydney 1902.* Legislative Assembly of N.S.W. Papers, 1902. Government Printer, Sydney.

Baehrel, R. 1950. Épidémie et terreur: Histoire et sociologie. *Annales Histoire Revolution Française* 22:113–46.

REFERENCES

Bailey, N.T.J. 1975. *The mathematical theory of infectious diseases and its applications.* C. Griffin, London.

Benevolent Society of New South Wales. 1839–51. List of diseases treated. *Annual reports.* Sydney. [ML]

Board of Health. 1881–2. *Instructions for Ambulance Corps.* Sydney.

———. 1883. *Report upon the late epidemic of smallpox 1881–1882.* Legislative Assembly of N.S.W. Papers. Government Printer, Sydney. 13 March.

Bouthoul, G., and R. Carrère. 1976. *Le défi de la guerre.* Presses Universitaires, Paris.

Boycott, J.A. 1971. *Natural history of infectious disease.* Edward Arnold, London.

Brownlea, A.A. 1972. Modelling the geographic epidemiology of infectious hepatitis. In N.D. McGlashan (ed.), *Medical geography,* 297–300. Methuen, London.

Burnet, F.M., and E. Clark. 1942. *Influenza: A survey of the last 50 years.* Macmillan, Melbourne.

Burnet, F.M., and D.O. White. 1972. *Natural history of infectious disease.* Cambridge University Press, Cambridge.

Butlin, N. 1983. *Our original aggression: Aboriginal populations of southeastern Australia 1788–1850.* Allen and Unwin, Sydney.

Chapin, C.V. 1925. Measles in Providence, R.I. *American Journal of Hygiene* 5:635–55.

Chevalier, L. 1958. *Le cholera, la premier épidémie du XIX siècle.* La Roche sur Yon.

Clark, R. 1981. *The journal and letters of Lt. Ralph Clark,* Fidlow and Ryan, Sydney.

Cleland, J.B. 1911. A contribution to the history of disease in Australia. *Australasian Medical Congress,* 9th session: 234–47.

———. 1914. Some diseases peculiar to, or of interest in, Australia. In J.H.L. Cumpston, *The history of smallpox in Australia, 1788–1908,* 163–70. Commonwealth Dept of Health, Government Printer, Melbourne.

Cliff, A.D., P. Haggett, J.K. Ord and G.R. Versey. 1981. *Spatial diffusion: An historical geography of epidemics in an island community.* Cambridge University Press, Cambridge.

Cobley, John. 1962. *Sydney Cove 1788.* Angus and Robertson, Sydney

———. 1963. *Sydney Cove 1789–1790.* Angus and Robertson, Sydney.

Collins, D. 1971. *An account of the English colony in New South Wales.* Reprint, Library Board of Sth Aust., Adelaide. Originally published London 1798, 1802.

Cooper, D.B. 1965. *Epidemic disease in Mexico City 1761–1813.* University of Texas Press, Austin.

Coulter, J. 1916. *Randwick Asylum: A historical review of the Society for the Relief of Destitute Children.* Sydney.

Creighton, C. 1965. *A history of epidemics in Britain,* vol. 2. Frank Cass, London. Originally published London 1894.

Cumpston, J.H.L. 1914. *The history of smallpox in Australia, 1788–1908.* Commonwealth Dept of Health, Government Printer, Melbourne.

———. 1919. *Influenza and maritime quarantine in Australia.* Commonwealth Dept of Health, Government Printer, Melbourne.

———. 1927. *The history of diphtheria, scarlet fever, measles and whooping cough in Australia, 1788–1925.* Commonwealth Dept of Health, Government Printer, Melbourne.

———. 1931. Public health in Australia. Part 1: The first forty-two years; Part 2: The second period, 1830 to 1850; Part 3: Developments after 1850. *Medical Journal of Australia* 1(17):491–500; 1(20):591–7; 1(23):679–85.

———. 1932. The evolution of public health administration in Australia. *Medical Journal of Australia* 1:194–8.

Cumpston, J.H.L., and F. McCallum. 1926. *The history of plague in Australia 1900–1925.* Commonwealth Dept of Health, Government Printer, Melbourne.

———. 1927. *The history of the intestinal infections (and typhus fever) in Australia 1788–1923.* Commonwealth Dept of Health, Government Printer, Melbourne.

Cunningham, P. 1966. *Two years in New South Wales*. Reprint, Angus and Robertson, Sydney. Originally published London 1827.

Director-General of Public Health. 1899, 1900, 1901. *Annual report of the Medical Officer of Health for the years 1898, 1899, 1900*. Government Printer, Sydney.

————. 1917. Outbreak of mild smallpox in Sydney and New South Wales 1913–16. (W.G. Armstrong). *Report of the Director-General of Public Health 1913–17*. Government Printer, Sydney.

————. 1920. Report on the influenza epidemic in New South Wales in 1919. In *Report of the Director-General of Public Health, N.S.W. for the year end 31 December 1919*. Government Printer, Sydney.

Dixon, C.W. 1962. *Smallpox*. J. & A. Churchill, London.

Donovan, J.W. 1970. Measles in Australia and New Zealand, 1834–1835. *Medical Journal of Australia* 1:5–10.

Eversley, D.E.C. 1965. Epidemiology as social history. In C. Creighton, *A history of epidemics in Britain*, Vol. 1, 3–39. Frank Cass, London.

Gandevia, B. 1971. Occupation and disease in Australia since 1788. Parts 1, 2. *Bulletin of the Post-graduate Committee in Medicine, University of Sydney* 27(8):157–97; 27(9):199–228.

————. 1978. *Tears often shed: Child health and welfare in Australia from 1788*. Pergamon, Sydney.

Gandevia, B., and J. Cobley. 1974. Mortality at Sydney Cove 1788–1792. *Australian and New Zealand Journal of Medicine* 4:111–25.

Gilder, G.A. 1938. The 'Faraway' and the smallpox outbreak of 1881–1882. *Journal and Proceedings Royal Australian Historical Society* 24:225–8.

Gladesville Asylum. 1892. *Report of the Inspector-General of the Insane 1891*. Government Printer, Sydney.

Gordon, D. 1976. *Health, sickness and society*. University of Queensland Press, St Lucia.

Haggett, P. 1972. Contagious processes in a planar graph: An epidemiological application. In N.D. McGlashan (ed.), *Medical geography*, 307–24. Methuen, London.

Ham, B. Burnett, 1907. *Report on plague in Queensland 1900–1907*. Queensland Dept of Public Health, Government Printer, Brisbane.

Health Society of New South Wales. 1876. *Hints for the prevention of scarlet fever*. John Sands, Sydney.

Hirst, L.F. 1953. *The conquest of plague*. Clarendon Press, Oxford.

Historical Records of Australia [*HRA*]. 1914–15. Series I, Vols 1–4. Government Printer, Sydney.

Historical Records of New South Wales [*HRNSW*]. 1892. Vol. 1, Part 2. Government Printer, Sydney.

Hocken, T.M. 1898. *Contributions to the early history of New Zealand (Otago)*. Low Marston, London.

Hollingsworth, T.H. 1979. A preliminary suggestion for the measurement of a mortality crisis. In H. Charbonneau and A. Larose (eds), *The great mortalities: Methodological studies of demographic crises in the past*, 21–8. Ordina, Leige.

Hughes, W.M. 1900. *New South Wales Parliamentary Debates*, Vol. 103. Government Printer, Sydney.

Hunter, J. 1968. *An historical journal of the transactions at Port Jackson and Norfolk Island*. Reprint, Library Board of Sth Aust., Adelaide. Originally published London 1793.

Jamieson, J. 1908. Periodicity in epidemic diseases. *Australasian Medical Congress*, 8th Session (2):97–103.

Langer, W.L. 1958. The next assignment. *American Historical Review* 63(2):283–304.

Lewis, M. 1980. *Milk, mothers and infant welfare*. In J. Roe (ed.), *Twentieth century Sydney*, 193–207. Hale and Iremonger, Sydney.

McGrew, R.E. 1965. *Russia and the cholera 1823–1832*. University of Wisconsin Press, Madison.

REFERENCES

Maclean, F.S. 1964. *Challenge for health: A history of public health in New Zealand.* Government Printer, Wellington.

Momiyama, M., and K. Katayama. 1966. A medico-climatological study in the seasonal variation of mortality in the United States of America. *Papers in Meteorology and Geophysics* 17(4):279–80.

Morley, D. 1980. Severe measles. In N.F. Stanley and R.A. Joske (eds), *Changing disease patterns and human behaviour,* 116–28. Academic Press, London.

Morrill, R.L., and J.J Angulo. 1979. Spatial aspects of a smallpox epidemic in a small Brazilian city. *Geographical Review* 69:319–30.

Parsons, H.F. 1970. *Report on the influenza epidemic of 1889–90* and *Further report and papers on epidemic influenza, 1889–92.* British Parliamentary Papers: Health and Infectious Diseases, Vol. 8, 1887–94:1–15, 318–24, 721–88. Irish University Press, Shannon.

Pollitzer, R. 1954. *Plague.* WHO, Geneva.

Pyle, G.F. 1969. The diffusion of cholera in the United States in the nineteenth century. *Geographical Analysis* 1:59–75.

Ray, A. 1976. The diffusion of diseases in the western interior of Canada, 1830–1850. *Geographical Review* 66(2):139–57.

Razzell, P. 1977. *The conquest of smallpox.* Caliban Books, Firle, Sussex.

Registrar-General. 1858–1901. Vital Statistics. *Annual report of the Registrar-General transmitting abstracts of marriages, births and deaths,* 1857–1900. Legislative Assembly of N.S.W. Papers, 1858–1901.

Roe, M. 1976. Smallpox in Launceston, 1887 and 1903. *Papers and Proceedings Tasmanian Historical Research Association* 23:111–48.

Rosen, G. 1967. People, disease and emotion: Some newer problems for research in medical history. *Bulletin of the History of Medicine* 41:5–23.

Royle, H.G. 1973. The state of health in New South Wales in the 1820s. *Medical Journal of Australia* 1:950–3.

Scarlet Fever. 1876. *Prevention of scarlet fever. Memorandum of Acting Medical Adviser to the Government.* Legislative Assembly of N.S.W. Papers, 1875–6, Vol. 6. Government Printer, Sydney.

Sewage and Health Board. 1876. *Report of the committee appointed by the Sydney City and Suburban Sewage and Health Board, 8th report.* Legislative Assembly of N.S.W. Papers, 1875–6, Vol. 5. Government Printer, Sydney.

Stock, R.F. 1976. *Cholera in Africa.* International African Institute, London.

Sydney Dispensary. 1828–45. List of diseases treated. *Annual reports.*

Sydney Dispensary and Infirmary. 1845–82. List of diseases treated. *Annual reports.*

Tench, W. 1979. *Sydney's first four years.* Reprint, Library of Australian History, Sydney. Originally published, *A complete account of the settlement at Port Jackson,* London 1793.

Thomas, D.J. 1867. On the recent epidemic in Melbourne of measles, scarlet fever and rubeola. *Transactions Medical Society of Victoria* 12:83–92.

Tidswell, F. 1898. A brief sketch of the history of smallpox and vaccination in New South Wales. *Australasian Association for the Advancement of Science* 7:1058–66.

Vaccination, 1882. *Meeting of Cabinet — Opinions upon compulsory vaccination.* Legislative Assembly of N.S.W. Papers, 1881. Government Printer, Sydney.

Watson, J.F. 1911. *The history of Sydney Hospital from 1811 to 1911.* Government Printer, Sydney.

Wentworth, W.C. 1820. *A statistical, historical and political description of the colony of New South Wales.* W.B. Whittaker, London.

———. 1824. *A statistical account of the British settlements in Australasia,* Vol. I. G.B. Whittaker, Sydney.

White, J. 1790. *Journal of a voyage to New South Wales.* J. Debrett, London.

Willey, K. 1979. *When the sky fell down.* Collins, Sydney.

Wilson, R.T. 1927. Annual report of the Central Board of Health of Victoria, 1875. In J.H.L. Cumpston, *The history of diphtheria, scarlet fever, measles and whooping cough in*

Australia, 1788–1925, 350–8. Commonwealth Dept of Health, Government Printer, Melbourne.

Young, C.M. 1979. Epidemics of infectious diseases in Australia prior to 1914. In H. Charbonneau and A. Larose (eds), *The great mortalities: Methodological studies of demographic crises in the past*, 207–27. Ordina, Leige.

Index